The Problem Orientated
Medical Record

Forward.
P 38

The Problem Orientated Medical Record (POMR)

ITS USE IN HOSPITALS, GENERAL PRACTICE AND MEDICAL EDUCATION

EDITED BY

J. C. Petrie M.R.C.P.

Senior Lecturer in Therapeutics and Clinical Pharmacology,
University of Aberdeen

Neil McIntyre M.D., F.R.C.P.

Reader in Medicine, Royal Free Hospital and
School of Medicine, London

FOREWORD BY

Sir Francis Avery Jones

CHURCHILL LIVINGSTONE
EDINBURGH LONDON AND NEW YORK 1979

CHURCHILL LIVINGSTONE
Medical Division of Longman Group Limited

Distributed in the United States of America by
Longman Inc., 19 West 44th Street, New York,
N.Y. 10036, and by associated companies,
branches and representatives throughout
the world.

First published 1979

ISBN 0 443 01405 1

British Library Cataloguing in Publication Data
The problem orientated medical record.
  1. Medical records.
  I. Petrie, J C   II. McIr tyre, N
  651.5   R864   78–40709

Printed in Hong Kong by
Sing Cheong Printing Co Ltd

Foreword

Medical records are important. Their function is primarily to assist clinical decision-making in diagnosis and treatment. They serve as an important means of communication of information between the clinical team treating the patient. They provide a discipline which plays an essential role in the education of medical students and junior doctors. They allow assessments to be made of the quality of medical care and provide data needed for the planning of health care services. They can play an important role in facilitating clinical and epidemiological research, and they provide evidence which may be essential for medico-legal purposes.

The need for better medical records has arisen for a number of reasons. Today, both in general practice and in hospitals, medical care relates less and less to one doctor. Clinical information must be available not only for other doctors but also, at least in part, to members of the team helping in the diagnosis and treatment. There is a much wider conceptual approach. There is much more information being made available and there is little point in this being so if such information is too difficult to retrieve from unorganized notes.

The problem has been building up imperceptibly in recent years and the need for a more systematic approach to the storing of information has become an urgent need. A sharp increase in the amount of clinical investigations now undertaken makes it all the more necessary to make certain that the patient gets the full benefit from them, and also, as spenders from the national purse, to assess the real contribution they make to better management of the patient's illness. Well-organized notes can not only be invaluable but interesting, stimulating, money-saving and educative. The student who qualifies, having learned to put down clinical information logically and simply, in a way that others can share, will become a much better doctor than those who become accustomed to scrappy, untidy notes. Already an appreciable number of doctors up and down the country, both in general practice and in hospitals, have gone to the trouble of reorganizing their notes. This book will be a great help in enabling others to follow their example.

One of the greatest pains to human nature is the pain of a new idea.
Walter Bagehot
I admit that the problem is a large and difficult one, but so are all problems until we begin to tackle them.
Sir Oliver Lodge
Of all work producing results nine-tenths must be drudgery.
Bishop Philpotts

1978   F.A.J.

Preface

There is growing interest in the problem-orientated medical record (POMR) and more widespread recognition of the potential for improving the quality of care given to patients. But in trying to apply POMR individuals run into difficulties; there are many reasons for this. We hope that the account of our experience of these real difficulties and the emphasis on important practical points will contribute to successful implementation of POMR in hospitals and general practice. We also hope that this book will help teachers to explore the enormous educational potential of POMR.

1978   J.C.P.
                                                                     N.Mc.I.

Contributors

S. V. Cantrill M.D.
PROMIS Laboratory, University of Vermont, Burlington, Vermont, U.S.A.

A. J. Hedley M.D., M.R.C.P.
Senior Lecturer in Community Health, University of Nottingham.

G. J. Lloyd B.Sc., M.R.C.P.
Lecturer, Academic Department of Medicine, Royal Free Hospital, London.

N. McIntyre M.D., F.R.C.P.
Reader in Medicine, Royal Free Hospital and School of Medicine, London.

J. C. Petrie M.R.C.P.
Senior Lecturer in Therapeutics and Clinical Pharmacology, University of Aberdeen, Honorary Consultant Physician, Aberdeen Teaching Hospitals.

M. G. Sheldon M.R.C.G.P.
General practitioner, Banbury, Oxon.

A. J. Tulloch M.D., F.R.C.G.P.
General practitioner, Bicester, Oxon; Research Assistant, Community Health Project, Unit of Clinical Epidemiology, University of Oxford.

Contents

1

The collection and utilisation of clinical information

A. J. HEDLEY

Senior Lecturer, Department of Community Health, University of Nottingham

INTRODUCTION

The purpose of this chapter is to discuss some of the general issues which doctors and other health professionals should consider when choosing and developing a method for the collection and utilisation of clinical information.

Texts on the history of medicine do not include any analysis of the development of clinical records. Yet many of us believe that good quality records are fundamental for sound clinical work. In Britain the introduction of the National Health Service led to obligatory record keeping (Cormack, 1971). Prior to that practitioners were only required to maintain records for patients' participation in insurance schemes and patient management often depended on recollections and not on records. Despite recent interest and innovation in medical record design and use, many of our records are chaotic repositories of information on which continuity of patient care is almost wholly dependent.

In contrast to progress in medical technology, there has been a notable lack of advancement in the techniques we use to document individual patient care. It is now almost 20 years since an expert committee urged improvement in the legibility of records (Ministry of Health, 1959). During this time, both the size and complexity of clinical records have increased. These factors constantly threaten to outstrip our capacity to control and use efficiently the information which our records contain.

It is surprising that the need for change was not anticipated when one considers the frustration, annoyance, confusion and inefficiency caused by voluminous and mainly unstructured patient records. There is an urgent need for change and medical schools should recognise that one of their principal goals must be to train both teachers and their students to adopt a more rational and flexible approach to the task of documenting patients' problems. It is also reasonable to expect all professional health workers to use social, clinical and laboratory information about their patients so that at the very least no harm is done. This is an issue which assumes greater importance when it is recognised that the patient's record, which was once the preserve of clinicians – if not one individual – may now carry contributions from different doctors and several non-medical health personnel.

WHY DO WE COLLECT AND RECORD CLINICAL INFORMATION?

Setting objectives

Any kind of organisation needs review and reassessment to ensure that its methods of working are appropriate to the functions which it serves. One way of promoting this process of review and reassessment is to set a standard or reference point against which the performance of the organisation can be measured. The first step in designing a record system is to reach agreement on a set of clearly defined objectives which would be accepted by teachers and other clinicians, by students and by other health personnel. One such set of objectives for constructing and maintaining records was suggested by McIntyre (1974) (Tables 1.1 and 1.2).

Table 1.1 Uses of medical records

1. Detailed reminder of clinical and laboratory information and therapy
2. Source of information about past illnesses and treatment
3. Facilitate continuity of care when several doctors involved
4. Assist evaluation and planning of health care system
5. Clinical research
6. Medical education
7. Audit of medical care
8. Litigation

Table 1.2 Principles of information retrieval from medical records

1. Record must be available
2. Its information must be
   a. Understandable (legibility, language)
   b. Correct and in context
   c. Adequate
3. To be able to find and assimilate this information quickly we must
   a. Use a standard structure
   b. Emphasise key points
   c. Reduce bulk by
      (i) Avoiding unnecessary entries
      (ii) Condensing without loss of information (laboratory records, précis of notes)

Construction and use of records

There is a surprisingly wide variation in what different doctors expect from the patient record. Some doctors want to see the record before making a diagnosis and treating a new patient; others it seems do not because they proceed without reference to it (Department of Health and Social Security, 1971).

Methods of archiving cumulative profiles of patients are still far from satisfactory, and vary between individuals, specialties and hospitals. Doctors are not good at routine tasks such as abstracting and summarising. It may be that their deployment in this way is unnecessary and that specially trained lay people should be used, but clearly doctors *must* first establish workable guidelines based on the need for specific types of clinical information.

The standardisation of records, for example by using pre-printed proformas and check-lists has both supporters and opponents. The latter claim that an individualistic approach to medicine is inhibited and that such forms may provide misleading indicators that a particular test or examination had been completed. Any system is open to misuse or abuse but the opponents of standardisation in medical records must demonstrate that the criteria of thoroughness and reliability are satisfied by records which are open-ended and of variable format. The danger that the process of medical enquiry might be inhibited by standardisation must be acknowledged but surely attempts should be made now to agree on the minimum essential information required to construct a basic patient record.

It is also now important that all health personnel should recognise and understand the need for a *system* of information collection, analysis and feedback in which each of the several million medical records held by the National Health Service is an important and integral part. In attempting to frame an acceptable set of objectives for the collection of clinical information we are confronted with perhaps the most contentious issue in this discussion. If the health services are to derive maximum benefit from the information resource represented by individual patients and their medical records, all health professionals must recognise and accept that the potential value of their own records extends beyond the horizons of the general practice surgery, hospital ward or outpatient clinic.

The factors which must be taken into account in creating and using a medical record include:

1. Need to provide individual patient care
2. Needs of patients as consumers
3. Needs of professional health personnel
4. Need to measure and evaluate health care

Obviously our objectives in the creation and utilisation of medical records can and should be set at several different levels. At the same time we require a unifying principle to encompass all of them. That principle is determined by the necessity for a system of record keeping which first meets our immediate needs for patient care, second provides clinical information which can be studied using epidemiological methods, and third is sufficiently flexible to accommodate changing needs and patterns of practice.

In the following sections several questions are addressed to the reader in an attempt to illustrate the central role of the medical record in health care and to emphasise that, for most of us, our present concept of the scope and potential of the medical record, its construction and its use, is far too limited.

NEED TO PROVIDE INDIVIDUAL PATIENT CARE

This is our first priority. It must not be compromised by any of the other requirements of the medical record system. The procedures and devices which can be employed to create a dynamic case record are described in detail elsewhere in this volume but here I challenge the health professional! Is the information he or she collects, and the way in which it is handled, the most appropriate for solving patients' problems and does it meet the wider requirements of a health service which has as its prime objectives, the promotion of health, prevention of disease and the delivery of continuous and comprehensive health care?

Reliability of clinical methods

The reliability of clinical methods, data and judgements has been the subject of scientific experiment and discussion for many years. There is a renaissance of interest in both the reliability and shortcomings of the methods we use to collect clinical information. Despite the importance of the history, the source of the information on which many diagnoses are based, there has been a conspicuous lack of effort to standardise such methods of collection. The need to do so has been demonstrated, for example, by wide disagreement, between different observers, in the prevalence ratios of symptoms in the same patient population. Fairbairn, Wood and Fletcher, (1959) used a questionnaire specifically designed to elicit respiratory symptoms. When the method of collecting the information is unstructured and 'open-ended', discrepancies are likely to be very much greater. Frequently agreement between clinicians working in the same clinical environment is no greater than would be expected by chance alone. This problem of disagreement between doctors is difficult to tackle in the context of routine clinical practice. It is clearly one of the most important factors influencing the content of a patient's medical record.

It must be emphasised that the quality of the information collected can be improved. Standard methods of collecting clinical information, relating to symptoms from different organs including cardiovascular (Rose and Blackburn, 1968), respiratory, (Medical Research Council, 1966) gastro-intestinal, (Horrocks et al 1976) and locomotor systems (Ritchie et al 1968) and endocrine glands (Crooks, Murray and Wayne, 1959; Crooks, Wayne and Robb, 1960; Billewicz et al 1969; Gurney et al 1970) have been designed, tested and validated by several groups of workers. These studies have helped to improve diagnostic methods by identifying those symptoms which are the *best* discriminants between patients who have or have not got the disease in question. The ability to produce, or at least support a selective diagnosis in this way creates opportunities for reducing the number of additional investigations which are needed for satisfactory patient management. 'Test reduction', it need hardly be said has important economic implications. Many of these standardised validated methods of clinical enquiry include, in addition to symptoms, the recognition and recording of specific physical signs and there are many more studies which demonstrate both intra and inter-observer variation for procedures in a routine physical examination (Koran, 1975).

Several authors have demonstrated that a critical review of clinical outcome in the light of the information originally collected at the first contact with the patient may lead to revision of the content of standard data collection forms and observational criteria and, as a consequence, improvement in performance.

Influence of records on the quality of individual patient care

A convincing demonstration is needed that both the design of the medical record and the methods used to complete it have a direct influence on our ability to deliver high quality care to individual patients. Many of the advantages of a structured standard record are self-evident but evaluation of its use in the management of specific clinical problems is often difficult and inconclusive. However, although there are inevitably instances where the method of documenting the *process* of care has minimal impact on *outcome*, this is certainly not true for many acute and chronic clinical problems.

The need to provide blood-pressure surveillance and treatment, (at specified levels of diastolic and systolic pressure) for defined sections of the population, is now clearly evident from both epidemiological studies (Kannel and Dawber, 1974) and actuarial data (Society of Actuaries, 1959). Ongoing studies aim to determine the level of 'cut-off' points for treatment (Blackburn, 1973; Medical Research Council, 1977). Hypertension exemplifies the importance of the medical record in case-finding; it provides a crucial link between a statement of intent (eg. to provide blood-pressure surveillance) and the achievement of anticipatory care. Heller and Rose, (1977a, 1977b) studied the recording of blood pressure in both hospital and general practice. They found that only 58 per cent of a random sample of all new patients attending two hospitals had a blood pressure recording in their notes and the figure was as low as 32 per cent for outpatient encounters. There were apparently no differences between the teaching and non-teaching hospital. Their studies suggest that hospitals are not acting effectively as centres for prevention and the medical record is not being used as a tool to promote comprehensive care. In general practice the proportion of records with completed blood pressure entries found by Heller and Rose ranged from 4 per cent to 36 per cent in five London general practice units, compared with 38 per cent in a random sample of nearly 3000 Scottish citizens and their general practice records. (Barlow *et al* 1977). These figures can be contrasted with Tudor Hart's (1970) demonstration that documentation of blood pressure can be achieved in virtually 100 per cent of the adult population at-risk within the context of routine general practice.

Dollery *et al* (1977) studied the performance of doctors using a structured record against those with a conventional 'open-ended' record. They showed, in a hypertension clinic, that performance in collecting relevant information including enquiry, clinical measurement and investigation was better with a structured record. It is disturbing that in both groups decisions on whether to collect information was often not related to a previously agreed clinical policy. 'Not recorded' does not necessarily mean 'not done', but failure to enter an important event into the progress notes or a summary document may lead directly to inadequate care, deterioration and readmission.

Medical records are also crucial in drug therapy. They are the link between the decision to treat and the act of treatment. Many types of drug records and different methods of using them have been tried in everyday hospital practice. Their inadequacies have become much more important with the increasing availability of potent therapeutic agents.

Crooks, Calder and Weir (1967) compared prescriptions on treatment records with the medicine lists used by nurses to administer the individual doses. There was a one in five variation between what the doctor had intended and what the nurses had transcribed to their medicine lists. The implications of such deficiencies in recording procedures, in terms of patient care, were obvious as was the need for improved drug documentation. Crooks *et al* (1965) developed a prescribing system which, used correctly, eliminates transcribing errors and minimises those of interpretation: The system has been shown to be valuable and to be acceptable under routine clinical conditions.

The fact that a prescription is legible and instructions clear does not of course give any indication as to whether the drug has been administered, so a simple, accurate and quick method of recording administration was devised (Crooks *et al* 1967). Initially, nurses were apprehensive about the introduction of yet another record but soon found that it made a useful contribution to patient management.

Education is not enough on its own; we need in addition some form of omnipresent guidance system such as the one described above for clinical practice. The very least it will allow us to achieve is a better understanding of what it is we do under the usual conditions of clinical practice.

Collection of clinical information and the prevention of errors in clinical practice

Macdonald (1976) has emphasised our fallability in the collection and interpretation of important clinical information. He showed that standardising the documentation of patient information may not in itself ensure that clinical care is of a high standard (set against agreed criteria) and consistently free from avoidable errors. Macdonald also showed that the effectiveness of a record derived from a pre-agreed protocol was increased when it was combined with computer-generated signals designed to draw attention to coincident events of clinical importance such as the administration of digoxin in the presence of a rising blood urea. The fact that computing technology was employed in this study should not obscure the finding that even good clinicians have major limitations in their capacity to process the information in a patient record and cannot consistently anticipate and avoid predictable adverse combinations of clinical, pathological and therapeutic events which may have serious implications for the patient.

All the doctors participating in the study accepted and acted on recommendations from the computer held protocols. They responded to a far greater extent than when such recommendations were not offered during control periods. Nevertheless as in the trial conducted by Dollery et al (1977) Macdonald showed that, despite indicating in writing that a particular course of action is required, in practice doctors frequently omit it or do something else!

When it is pointed out that clinicians have failed to comply with pre-agreed criteria they usually respond by questionning the criteria rather than considering of ways of improving performance. It is obviously important that we should learn more about behavioural patterns of this kind – a task which will only be possible by using a purpose designed system and previously agreed explicit protocols for patient care.

There is also much evidence that 'traditional' records do not function well as long term support systems for the surveillance of chronic disease. *Intended* medication in many different clinical problems is frequently not taken (Dixon, Stradling and Wooton, 1957; Joyce, 1962; Porter, 1969; Willcox, Gillan and Hare, 1965; Bonnar, Goldberg and Smith, 1969). Another source of errors in clinical practice arises from failure to transfer information about current drug therapy to patients or to other clinicians. In one study (Beveridge and Petrie, 1972) no information was available from medical sources about 1002 (64 per cent) of a total of 1557 drugs taken by 498 patients referred to hospital. 613 (61 per cent) of the 1002 drugs for which information was lacking (mainly hypnotics, sedatives and analgesics) were supplied by prescription. The implications of such poor communication are considerable. For example in another study (Seidl et al 1966) almost half of the adverse reactions to drugs prescribed in hospital occurred in the first three days – and particularly during the first twenty-four hours. We have had this kind of evidence for a long time but have failed to appreciate the extent to which it negates the initial effort and enterprise in diagnosis and treatment.

Several studies on the prevention of errors in clinical practice emphasise that ignorance is not usually responsible for the errors of omission. Perhaps our methods of working are simply inadequate to cope with the number and volume of transactions which occur. More effective use should be made of the record to co-ordinate our activities and raise clinical practice to a uniform standard which is commensurate with existing knowledge. Smart (1975) has spelled out the implications for clinicians if we fail to develop a more systematic and thorough examination of our own daily professional activities. Without it we are vulnerable to unwanted and probably damaging sanctions and restrictions on clinical practice.

NEEDS OF PATIENTS AS CONSUMERS

Acquisition of medical knowledge by patients

'Not to be handled by the patient' is an old caveat but one which is still being printed on the covers of medical records. It contrasts with the growing demand from patients for greater participation in certain aspects of their medical management and better access to and ownership of medical knowledge and clinical information relating to the health problems of individual patients. There may be several reasons for this, including higher levels of secondary education and continuing change in social attitudes and policies.

Medical knowledge should not be the preserve of the professions. Such elitism is unfashionable and unwanted. Doctors and other health personnel should be the prime movers in bringing about a change of attitudes and practice. Firstly patients have a right to know about and to understand their health problems and their practitioners' interpretation of them. The transmission of the contents of the medical record in the form of a summary of current problems and management plans is not easy, and some patients may not wish to have it, while others may react adversely to this knowledge. Nevertheless neither of these difficulties is a valid reason for opposition to the basic principle. Secondly no doctor can solve all his patients' problems and he will certainly not always be present to discuss and explain his own findings on each occasion when this is necessary. For example locums may do night calls or patients may be taken to an accident and emergency department. Therefore it is the patient's record and particularly crucial parts of it – such as the problem list and treatment record –

which should form a continuum throughout the patient's life. This is invariably not the case with his or her medical attendants.

Most medical consultations occur in general practice, key decisions are made, including identification of main problems, referral for secondary care and admission to hospital. Contacts with the practitioner provide the main opportunities for prevention. Errors of omission must be regarded as a form of iatrogenic disease so long as we fail to seek new ways of using the record to prevent their occurrence.

The contribution of patients to clinical information in their medical record

Many doctors are pessimistic about the feasibility of educating patients about their health problems, for example in the area of chronic disease, to the extent that they could begin to participate more effectively in their own management. Some doctors believe that the level of 'intelligence' and 'education' of their patients are insuperable impediments to progress. However several studies have shown that patients can help health personnel to collect information effectively. Indeed our patients may represent the greatest paramedical force within the health service (Weed, 1973). However, in the United Kingdom, the idea that the patient can help remains, with one or two notable exceptions, largely untried and untested. The concept that patients can both contribute directly to and utilise the information held in their record has so far gained little acceptance – at least there is little tangible evidence of it. What is needed is the creation of a system in which such ideas can be tested. One glance at the narrative of an unstructured in-patient record and the random jottings generated in out-patient clinics will be sufficient to convince the majority that our patients cannot join us if we continue to use our present methods of record-keeping.

We also need properly designed studies to evaluate patient education programmes by means of *pre-* and *post-hoc* observations on test groups using different instructional techniques. In one such exercise with patients with rheumatoid disease (Vignos, Parker and Thompson, 1976) whose characteristics (educational level, intellectual function, socio-economic status) were defined by standard tests and measures, a programme of carefully prepared reading material, reinforced by illustrated lectures led to a marked improvement in patients' understanding of their health problem, as measured by pre- and post-testing using a multiple choice questionnaire. Although existing knowledge correlated with previous educational attainment and socio-economic status, the post-instructional improvement did not.

Patient completed questionnaires

Tait and Stevens (1973) advocated methods of completing essential baseline information in the medical record – either in the surgery or clinic or at home without necessarily the participation of a doctor. Sheldon's (1976) study provides a striking demonstration of the range and depth of relevant information which patients may provide when given the opportunity to express themselves using a questionnaire which includes open-ended responses. It recalls Rene Laennec's exhortation 'Listen to your patient! He is giving you the diagnosis' (Hodgkins, 1965). Laennec died in 1826 but we have hardly exploited his idea in the intervening years.

Self-administered clinical questionnaires have been used to initiate or update the clinical record in general practice by Bjorn and Cross (1970) in the USA and by Lefever and his colleagues in the UK (Lefever, West and Trevelyan, 1977). Reports by Anderson and Day (1968), Hall (1972) and Gumpel and Mason (1974) describe similar studies in medical out-patient departments. Gumpel and Mason suggested that the recorded information might form part of the data base for a problem orientated record.

A two stage questionnaire has been successfully introduced into a gynaecology clinic (Robinson *et al* 1975). In the 'root' questionnaire the patient indicates the problem area and additional information is collected by means of an appropriate 'branch' questionnaire. The authors found a high level of patient acceptance and showed that, particularly in a sensitive area of clinical practice concerned with sexual behaviour and fertility, the questionnaires provided an effective interface with the patient. They generated good quality clinical information which achieved a higher level of comprehensive coverage than conventional unstructured histories obtained from patients with similar age, social class and gynaecological problems.

The need for sound and comprehensive methods of collecting baseline clinical information is nowhere more important than in the health care of the aged. A complex mixture of social, economic and medical factors must be noted, distilled and assessed. Hall (1974) emphasised the need to use multiple sources of information in assessing the problems of the elderly. Many previous studies have demonstrated the need to provide anticipatory care for populations of apparently well old people. When previously unreported (or un-recorded) illness has been sought by multi-disciplinary teams a high prevalence of serious problems, which were susceptible to treatment, was found in 20 per cent to 30 per cent of those interviewed and examined. In one study Williamson *et al* (1964) were concerned at the advanced state of the physical and mental problems in patients admitted to the wards. They expressed the view that general practitioners should maintain old-age registers and regular contact with the elderly. Within the framework of general practice the clinical team must accept responsibility for comprehensive care of a defined population group and it should develop methods which will help it to deliver preventive medical care, treatment and patient education.

Many of the early programmes for screening and case-finding used practice nurses and health visitors to collect information and complete a socio-medical data base. The extent to which older members of a practice population can themselves contribute to the baseline information in their records has received little attention. Declining cognitive function and failing acuity in the special senses might be considered good reasons why older patients would not be able to participate in contributing to the initiation and maintenance of their medical record. One case study (Hedley and Ryan, 1977) illustrates that this is not necessarily true.

In a study of 307 elderly patients on the register of a new town health centre, 165 were offered an assisted interview to complete a data base comprising social, economic and health information and 142 received a self-administered document. There was no difference between the two target groups in the proportion who accepted the arrangements at the first request nor in the frequency of positive and negative responses in 85 per cent of the variables included in the data base. The results are encouraging and indicate the need for further studies on the utility of this approach to the completion of background information for anticipatory medical care.

Objections raised against self-administered questionnaries as methods of collecting basic clinical information include:

1. Failure of patients to complete long documents.
2. Difficulties for the clinician in analysing and assimilating the information.
3. Interference with the doctor/patient relationship.

However, it is clear from reported studies that patient compliance is good. Information from well designed questionnaires allows the identification of relevant problems and allows clinicians to spend more time on them. Many patients have expressed a preference for questionnaires as a method of first contact. Anderson and Day found that only 7 per cent of responses were unsatisfactory and that in a further 5.6 per cent the patients were illiterate or could not read

English. There will undoubtedly be cultural and geographical differences, initially, in the acceptance of methods which enable patients to contribute directly to their medical records but there is no evidence that achieving a satisfactory interface between patient, medical record and doctor is beyond our wit and ingenuity.

Retention and use of medical records by patients

To be really effective in ensuring quality and continuity in medical care, medical records must be both complete and available at the time of consultation. Hospitals frequently fall short of these requirements. The time for retrieval of records for new admissions varies from ten minutes to as long as two days (Department of Health and Social Security, 1971), particularly if records have to be transferred between hospitals. In one department of obstetrics and gynaecology, 300 records had to be retrieved for one day's outpatient sessions (Murray and Topley, 1974). After defining the needs of patients, doctors, midwives and clerical staff, this group chose to give the complete obstetric hospital record to the patient. Their experience with this experiment is impressive. A total of 10,000 records were carried, only two were irretrievably lost – an enviable performance in any context! A saving of 1750 hours of clerical time (for pulling and re-filing notes) and 315 of audio-typing was achieved. Acceptance by both patients and general practitioners was uniformly high. There are therefore many reasons why the patient could act as an appropriate and highly motivated custodian of their medical record; increasing acceptance of this approach would provide a very effective means of promoting patient education.

The continual exchange of information between general practitioner, patient and specialist is an essential feature of the management of chronic disease when care is shared between two or more clinicians. A community care service for diabetics originally developed by a hospital based diabetic clinic (Hill, 1976) recognised the importance of good communications to promote integration of diabetic care. In addition to recommendations on management to general practitioners, advice to patients is offered in the form of a patient held document, designated a 'co-operation record book'. At each patient encounter with community nurse, health visitor or doctor in general practice or hospital clinics, an entry describing the patient's clinical status, diet, insulin and oral hypoglycaemic therapy can be made. The co-operation record book for diabetic patients developed by these workers has now been made widely available by an independent organisation (Hoechst Meducation Service, 1976).

THE NEEDS OF PROFESSIONAL HEALTH WORKERS

Clinical research

Most clinicians have difficulty in assessing and using their own accumulated experience in the management of patients with specific conditions. Clinical research is often a tedious process of abstraction from open-ended records by different authors with varying amounts of unstructured narrative and laboratory results. There are problems in nosology and therefore in identifying groups of patients with similar characteristics, in handling groups of data with missing values and in analysis and interpretation. We have developed a high level of tolerance to this form of imprecision. To adopt alternative methods of working may not always be easy and for the individual to change may sometimes be very difficult. There are several recent reports of attempts to achieve simple low-cost manual methods of data recording and collation, for clinical practice. The effectiveness of some of these procedures remains to be worked out. However, it is certain that health professionals will experience increasing difficulty in justifying casual and innumerate methods of collecting and processing information; good information is vital for clinical research, continuing education and evaluation of care.

In 1966 Small wrote '*Living Records*', an elegant and comprehensive account of the information needs of the clinician who wishes to apply an analytical approach to his clinical records. He squarely places the culpability for failing to design adequate records on the shoulders of the clinician.

Most routine clinical records are unusable as a basis for high quality clinical research. Research workers are usually obliged to use separate specially designed documents for data collection. This is also necessary when the information would not be documented in the normal course of patient care. However, when the information should have been recorded unnecessary duplication of effort and waste of resources occur – which could be avoided if the format of the record was standard and its obligatory content appropriate. Clinicians who wish to document, analyse and evaluate the care they provide, must establish special registers and information systems (Brooke, 1974; Hedley, 1977). Unfortunately some registers have been abandoned and discontinued because the information they hold is incomplete, inaccurate, or for other reasons unusable as a basis for clinical or operational research. Indeed these registers have frequently been condemned as a research tool on the basis of the second rate information which they provide. This problem has frequently been caused by the application of the same 'non-system' which currently prevails in conventional medical record keeping.

Although the potential rewards of research may stimulate some doctors to develop special record systems few doctors are sufficiently interested in the wider aspects of health care to be motivated to innovate in medical records and to continue to do so in response to changing demands and priorities in medical care.

Manpower planning and the collection of clinical information

The availability and deployment of personnel and resources are crucial factors in the planning and delivery of health care. There is now widespread interest in the concept that non-medical health personnel (NMHP) can be employed in new and extended clinical roles. Various terms have been used to describe the role of NMHP in different clinical situations – such as medical auxiliary, paramedical, physicians' assistants, nurse practitioners and nursing care specialists. Their actual roles may be very different, depending on the level of their general and professional education and experience – but it is the need to develop techniques to train them and evaluate their effectiveness which presents the really exciting challenge. Many consider that there is no longer any argument as to whether NMHP should be participating in the collection and use of clinical information, in both primary and secondary care (Backett and England, 1975). Those who accept the fundamental philosophy of 'needs-related' manpower planning will concur with this. The need for rapid and effective diversification in the roles of all health personnel has been quickly recognised in third world countries. Here the size of the problem of delivering basic health care, in the presence of severe economic constraints, highlights the shortfall which exists between manpower and the delivery of basic care when manpower planning is *only* related to the training of doctors; (Fendall, 1972; Morley, 1973; Mahler, 1974). Under the conditions of a randomised controlled trial (Spitzer *et al* 1974) the deployment of a nurse-practitioner has been shown to be cost-effective in that the patient groups (receiving traditional or mainly nurse-practitioner care) had a similar mortality experience and were comparable in terms of quality of care, physical, social and emotional indices and patient satisfaction.

Experiments on the collection and utilisation of clinical information by non-medical personnel have frequently been based on information from clinical and epidemiological studies, which has been incor-

porated into structured interviews, flowcharts and algorithms.*
Algorithms have been constructed for solving several clinical
problems for example, chest pain, fever, diarrhoea, sore throat,
urinary symptoms (Essex, 1976; O'Grady, Lambert and Begent,
1975; Sox, Sox and Tompkins, 1973) and for managing conditions
such as hypertension (Smith, 1975) and thyroid disease (Bayliss and
Hall) in different conditions of clinical practice (for example, primary
care, hospital out-patients, rural health care) in third world and
Western countries.

There are already important lessons to be learned by western health
care systems from innovations in the collection and utilisation of
clinical information in developing countries. The work of Essex (1976)
is an outstanding example of the way in which a multidisciplinary
approach to problem-solving for common clinical problems (in this
case in East Africa) can be both rationalised and revolutionised. He
summarises the principles of disease causation and control and
presents a series of algorithms for the diagnosis and management of
common health problems.

A systematic approach to problem solving is important because it
ensures prior agreement on the minimum amount of essential
information which must be collected in a given set of circumstances
and the way in which it must be handled. It allows the reliability of the
practitioner to be assessed and it may be used to identify where
deviations from the agreed plan occur. The development of these
techniques is an important discipline for all health professionals and
not least for doctors. This has been demonstrated in a gastroenterology
clinic where the collection of pre-defined data from patients by a
physician's assistant led to an improvement in the diagnostic
performance of clinicians who used this information later in a
conventional medical consultation (Horrocks and de Dombal, 1975).

In the case of hypertension, it is evident that if we are to achieve our
objective of documenting blood pressures of each member of the
population at risk then alternative strategies in the deployment of
manpower for the collection of clinical information are mandatory. In
the USA the Joint National Committee on Detection, Evaluation and
Treatment of High Blood Pressure (1977) emphasises the role of non-
physicians. All health care professionals should be strongly encouraged to take a patient's blood pressure routinely regardless of the

---

*The Algorithm is a method of plotting the strategy of problem-solving. The
method involves breaking down a problem so that every factor which determines
the solution can be represented as a separate question which can be answered in
terms of *Yes* or *No*. The logical interdependence of the questions can be indicated
in the form of a flowchart (Wheatley and Unwin, 1972).

reason for the patient's visit. If all existing health care facilities routinely offered blood pressure measurement the need for screening would diminish.

Diabetes is another clinical problem in which alternative plans for all aspects of continuing patient care are being studied. The work load is high in both young and old, in pregnant patients and in those with diabetic complications. Admissions to hospital for ketoacidotic coma is still a common event and diabetes is the commonest cause of blindness in British patients under age 50. The most important factor in achieving good control of diabetes, which the current evidence suggests will prevent microvascular complications leading to retinopathy, nephropathy and neuropathy (Cahill, Etzweiler and Freinkel, 1976) is the patient's expertise in managing their own disease. This in turn demands a high level of patient education, good communication between patient and practitioner and exchange of clinical information. To achieve this, experiments are in progress (Judd *et al* 1976) in which specialist nurses assume responsibility not only for continuity of care but also for first contact decisions when problems arise, and for supervision and patient education – especially of new diabetics. New methods of training are needed which will also allow performance to be monitored and properly evaluated. Without such developments there is a danger that opposition to extending the role of the nurse in this way (already apparent in some areas – British Medical Association, 1970, British Medical Association, 1977) may gain ground.

It is important that these studies, many of which have taken place overseas, are followed by firm action in British health care programmes. Statements of intent or at least encouragement are plentiful. The Royal College of General Practitioners (1973) has emphasised the need to define the type of health personnel required at first contact level, with a view to extending the roles of both non-medical personnel and general practitioners. A 1971 report on The Organisation of Group Practice (Central Health Services Council, 1971) firmly stated that much of the work undertaken by the GP could be delegated; a view also expressed by the present Minister of Health (Ennals, 1977). Extension of the role of the clinical nurse was envisaged in the Briggs report on nursing (Report of the Committee on Nursing, 1972) and increasing requests for guidance and advice on legal implications and training requirements have prompted the release of a definitive statement by the Department of Health and Social Security (1977).

Communication between health professionals: transfer of information from hospital to general practice

The management of patient problems should be viewed as an on-going process in which the central focus is the medical record. In the United Kingdom it is the general practice record which is the key to continuous care. Hospital care is episodic – often producing a limited and cross-sectional profile of a patient's problems at a particular point in time. Nevertheless, the hospital can and should provide an important form of support for the primary care services. Certainly the information acquired during a period of hospital care should be transferred to practice records in a form which allows maximum effective use. There is a good deal of evidence that this does not work well in practice. Heller and Rose (1977b) for example, found that when a high blood pressure *was* discovered in a hospital unit, the general practitioner was not informed in 22 per cent of cases.

In another study (Tulloch *et al* 1975) a group of general practitioners defined their information requirements and then assessed the extent to which these needs were met by discharge summaries from several hospital departments. Their results indicate large gaps in this method of communication between clinicians. Missing data was noted in the sections on patient identification information (patient's name, address, hospital number, date of birth, GP, hospital, department, consultant) clinical data (presenting symptoms, investigations, drugs, drug reactions, progress) and management (eg. future follow-up arrangements, prognosis and patient education). The authors found inordinate delays in the despatch of a discharge summary and the overall diagnostic assessment was not clear in 28 per cent of final reports. They emphasised the lack of a structured format in many records despite the superiority of structuring (for ease of reference) to free narrative. In designing medical records account must be taken of the needs of all health professionals who must use the clinical record in order to carry out their designated role effectively.

Medical records and continuing education

Despite our increasing awareness of the importance of achieving high standards of consistency and reliability in initiating and maintaining patient records – the allocation of curriculum time to this end, in medical schools, is generally an unusual event. The ability of the graduate to create and interpret a record is rarely tested and a similar lack of emphasis is placed on these skills in higher professional examinations, such as the MRCP. The collection and interpretation of clinical information in 'long' and 'short' cases is usually carried out before the examiner appears, a written record is not required and the candidate is assessed and may succeed even though he lacks these particular skills and competence. The problem of poor records is a recurring one and some form of non-punitive audit of the performance of all clinicians in constructing and using a patient record in problem solving is needed as part of the process of continuing education. Feinstein (1967) in his excellent monograph *Clinical Judgement* advocates direct monitoring of the process of acquiring clinical information. Weiner and Nathanson (1976) describe a method of achieving this within the context of routine clinical practice. They classify errors in completing the clinical examination into five categories.

1. Technique
2. Omissions
3. Detection
4. Interpretation
5. Recording

By ensuring that clinical rounds include a group assessment of the composition and logic of the record they demonstrate the potential for creating learning opportunities which are based on the medical record.

There has also been a marked increase in the number of independent learning methods and materials in response to the recognised need for better plans for continuing education and the relatively short half-life of clinical knowledge (Rosenow, 1971).

However, factual knowledge may not lead to an improvement in skills required for the collection and interpretation of clinical information. In the experience of one group (Ashbaugh and McKean, 1976), 55 group audit sessions covering 37 clinical problems and involving five and a half thousand records, showed that when deficiencies occurred, 94 per cent were in performance and only 6 per cent in factual knowledge. Poor record keeping is noted as a recurring problem but one which responds to the stimulus of scrutiny carried out along agreed guidelines in a non-punitive fashion.

NEED TO MEASURE AND EVALUATE MEDICAL CARE

Information for the management of clinical work in hospitals

Evaluation is concerned with setting objectives and determining whether those objectives are met. This approach results in the generation of questions about observed gaps between aims and achievements. Since the publication of the First Report of the Joint Working Party on the Organisation of Medical Work in Hospitals

(Ministry of Health, 1968) and its counterpart in Scotland (Scottish Home and Health Department, 1967) an increasing emphasis has been laid on the need for clinical consultants to participate in the management of specialist services and in so doing use statistical information derived from both their clinical activities and the population which they serve. To do this they must accept a large measure of responsibility for defining the data which should be collected and developing the mechanisms for its collection and eventual use. Our goal must be to progress to the stage where the management of clinical services includes the effective utilisation of good quality clinical information in such a way that we develop predictive tools, anticipate events and avoid breakdowns in services (Clayden and Metcalfe, 1977).

If clinicians were successful in this role then the expected result would be more rational determination of priorities in medical care and the better use and control of resources. However, decision making is difficult without good quality information and one reason why clinicians have so far largely failed to achieve an active part in management is that they are frustrated by lack of the information which they need to carry out this role effectively. Health statistics derived from clinical information are not custom-made for local management and many problems have been described in relation to their content and reliability; some of these are referred to in the following sections.

Records: the source of medical intelligence
We are all consciously or otherwise involved in activities which are aimed at improving our health care delivery system. Most of us are unaware of the possible use and importance of individual patient records in this process. In numerical terms the potential assets represented by clinical records are impressive. For example, in the Scottish Health Service, serving a population of around five million people, a year's work generates records from the following patient events (Bodenham and Wellman, 1972):

1. 650,000 admissions
2. 8 million attendances at outpatient departments
3. 28 million prescriptions
4. 2 million courses of dental treatment
5. 60,000 eye tests
6. 90,000 births
7. 60,000 deaths

This accumulated experience held in medical records is a valuable resource but we are only now beginning to study ways of utilising this

information more effectively – an activity which has in turn exposed
deficiencies in the methods used to collect it.

Clinical records and health information systems

The outcomes of several million episodes of illness (or manifestations
of disease) are now archived in information systems operated by
different offices of the state, for example, Hospital Activity Analysis
(HAA) (Morris *et al* 1974), Scottish Hospital In-Patient Statistics
(SHIPS) (Heasman, 1968) and the Registrar General's Causes of
Mortality. In each case the information catalogued has been generated
by a medical practitioner, but apart from the use of special senses and
the ability to write (not necessarily legibly) no other demands have
been made of practitioners. This is surprising in view of the enormous
resources applied to the task of collation and analysis of information
and its importance as an indicator of trends. It is truly ironical, when
one considers that doctors have been amongst the most vocal critics of
the inadequacies and inconsistencies of some of these systems, such as
those which feed back information based on hospital admissions.

No data collection system was generally applicable at the inception
of the National Health Service. The first of these, based on a form
designated SH3 (Department of Health and Social Security)
introduced in 1953, provided basic statistical data including bed
availability, occupancy and turnover, and numbers of discharges and
deaths. Work has been in progress for approximately 25 years to
develop a reliable system of documenting and summarising the clinical
outcome of episodes of hospital treatment. The objectives of this work
are to utilise patient information to derive both administrative and
clinical statistics for all professional health personnel and adminis-
trators.

The original system in England and Wales, implemented in 1950,
(Department of Health and Social Security) was designated the
Hospital In-Patient Enquiry (HIPE) and drew a 10 per cent sample of
hospital discharges including deaths in a calendar year; by 1957 it
covered all non-psychiatric hospitals. The further development of this
approach, HAA (Department of Health and Social Security, 1969) in
the 1960's, is aimed at total coverage of all hospital discharges. In
Scotland the Scottish Hospital In-Patient Statistics (SHIPS) has
provided 100 per cent coverage of discharges since 1961 (Scottish
Hospital In-Patient Statistics). The standard form used for data
collection carries information on patient identification, age, sex,
marital status, area of residence, admission and discharge as well as a
clinical summary including principal diagnoses and treatment. This
undertaking is a difficult, complex and expensive exercise but one

which may ultimately ensure that standardised methods of data collection, coding, analysis and record-linkage are applied to every patient record initiated in the ward or clinic. The absolute necessity for high quality patient records, which are the principal sources of this information, must be recognised if we are to make real progress in this field.

In opening their concise account of the development of HAA, Rowe and Brewer (1972) say that 'medical records must be improved in order that the service they provide will match the needs of modern medicine'. We must consider therefore to what extent our current medical records, as unique source documents are compatible with a standard national system. The question arises as to whether the methods and logic which have been employed to identify patients' problems are consistent with the goals of the systems which are being developed.

In 1969, the British Medical Association Planning Unit (British Medical Association Planning Unit, 1969; Heasman and Carstairs, 1971) commented on the 'unaccountable' variations in clinical management, using discharge summary data as their source. They produced evidence for a wide range of specific clinical problems treated in medical or surgical units; they demonstrated that duration of stay after admission, percentage of patients undergoing operations and interval between operation and discharge varied more than might have been anticipated and reflected large differences in resources consumed between different clinicians treating the same conditions. In Scotland, since 1969, data generated by clinical work has been used to provide feedback for consultants in the form of a confidential digest known as Scottish Consultant Review of In-Patient Statistics (SCRIPS) (Heasman, 1976). It provides information about the clinical activity of the consultant's unit including numbers of patients treated, diagnoses, outcome (discharge or death) and duration of stay. The majority of comments received from consultants in response to this form of feedback has been hostile. Many of them criticised errors and inconsistencies in the summary data. The following personal observation illustrates the kind of inconsistency encountered:

In a university teaching hospital medical unit, SCRIPS, in the form of a computer printed summary document, showed that more than 20 per cent of patients with a diagnostic label of hyperthyroidism were coded as 'thyrotoxicosis – without mention of goitre'. The figure was shown to be incorrect by re-examining a sample of the original patient records. This inconsistency arose because the listings of diagnoses in the medical records at that time were formulated in an arbitrary fashion and were incompatible with the adopted national system of coding and classifying morbidity and mortality using the WHO International Classification of Disease (ICD) (World Health Organisation, 1967).

The point is not that, in this particular instance anyone is necessarily blameworthy. We must acknowledge that our different information stores will continue to fail as providers of medical intelligence until *each stage* of the process of collection, coding and collation of clinical information is part of a purpose-designed system. Wilson (1976) reported that for a specific clinical problem, self-poisoning, transcription from the patient's medical record to the SHIPS coding document (SMR-1), was only correct in 77 per cent (which improved to 89 per cent two years later after this fact was publicised); in another hospital, it was only correct in 18 per cent and 64 per cent for the same two years. In discussing the reasons for dissatisfaction with SCRIPS, Heasman (1976) refers to the difficulty of 'abstracting from unclear or confusing records' and it is obvious that validity checks in computer programs will not improve the quality of information from records which are illogical or incomplete. It seems to be an unreasonable challenge to expect those responsible for preparing the input data to extract information from records with which, as clinicians, we ourselves often experience difficulties of interpretation. If a system such as SCRIPS is unreliable, this is because it is obliged to interface with a source document whose structure and content is uncertain and unreliable.

In the past it has been impossible to retrieve information about drugs prescribed and administered in hospital. The introduction of standardised drug recording procedures which have attained a high standard of legibility has made the routine retrieval of information from these records feasible.

The development of even a simple drug information system is a considerable task for a hospital discharging some 40,000 patients per annum since it has to cope with 150,000–200,000 prescriptions. Standardised recording procedures similar to the Aberdeen system were introduced in Dundee in 1971 and the two centres now have compatible files covering approximately 4300 beds, the file in 1977 comprised 400,000 patient discharges and approximately one and a half million prescriptions. Prescription data may be retrieved from duplicates of the standardised prescription records and linked to the patient identification and morbidity data recovered from the SMR-1 document to create a patient drug file.

The Aberdeen/Dundee medicines evaluation and monitoring

group drug file has mainly been used to aid investigations such as the follow-up of suspected adverse reactions. The file facilitates the immediate identification of all patients who have received a specific drug and it is subsequently possible to determine the number of patients exhibiting the suspected effect. It is also possible to determine the frequency with which similar events occur in suitably matched control populations not receiving the suspected drug, and thus confirm or refute suspected adverse reactions. The file can be used in the study of drug interactions and drug-disease interactions. Monitoring of new preparations is facilitated and the ability to identify large groups of patients receiving specific medication can be used to investigate drug efficacy. The system can also be used to study particular 'at risk' groups such as the elderly who may present special problems of efficacy and toxicity.

The file was originally developed to facilitate the investigation of adverse reactions but the information has been used to provide medical and nursing staff with information which might help in practical management and assessment of drug therapy. Bulletins giving information about differences which may have occurred between what the doctors prescribed and what the nurses recorded they had administered were found to be useful. Information about prescribing practices is readily available, reported differences in relation to patterns of drug-induced disease provoke new ideas and several clinicians have asked for further information. The provision of such information may have a role in continuing education and may go some way towards encouraging more rational and economic prescribing and thus make a contribution towards improving patient care.

There has been and perhaps still is, a nihilistic attitude towards this type of data collection in hospitals. Clinicians should acknowledge that the implementation of systems, such as SCRIPS, and the Aberdeen/ Dundee monitoring system has done a great deal to stimulate improvements in the collection and processing of clinical information by increasing awareness about our lack of proficiency in constructing medical records.

Death certification

This, the oldest form of statutory government statistic related to health care, is recorded by a medical practitioner and generated largely from information held in the patient's medical record, either in general practice or hospital. Some believe that death certificates are 'Not worth the paper they are written on' (*Lancet*, 1966). By contrast a distinguished epidemiologist (Doll, 1976) wrote that the Registrar General's record of causes of mortality 'has been one of Britain's most valuable contributions to world medicine . . . comparable with the introduction of vaccination against smallpox and the discovery of penicillin'. Undoubtedly the interpretation of secular trends in deaths from specific diseases – such as tuberculosis (decreasing) and lung cancer (increasing) has provided unique information about changes in mortality, their possible relationship to social and therapeutic intervention and about behavioural patterns in the population. In special studies however, death certificates have been found wanting in several respects. There may be at least two problems here. The first is that the process of care may not have provided sufficient information on which to base a reasonable classification of the cause(s) of death without further investigation by autopsy. But, how often do we make the best use of the record to seek indications for autopsy or even to rank the patient's problems so that the best summary of the patho-physiological processes leading to death is achieved? The second problem, of course, is that for many patients the case record is incapable of yielding the type of information which would allow reasonable certainty to be achieved in the coding of causes of death. The quality of the medical record must have an important bearing on the reliability of mortality statistics and there is clearly a case for assessing the contribution that can be made to their improvement by better problem identification. The General Register Office report (Heasman and Lipworth, 1966) on the accuracy of certification of causes of death revealed under-diagnosis in tuberculosis, dissecting and non-syphilitic aortic aneurysms and malignant tumours of brain, kidney, cervix, ovary, pancreas and biliary tract. Over-diagnosis occurred for pulmonary embolus, cerebral haemorrhage, infectious hepatitis and colonic carcinoma.

These comments largely apply to deaths occurring in hospitalised patients. Deaths occurring after discharge from hospital are of interest (or should be) to specialists as well as to the general practitioner responsible for the patients' management. In a review of the clinical significance of deaths occurring outside the hospital, one group of investigators (Rang, Acheson and O'Connor, 1968) found that some specialist and cottage hospitals did not keep records which were adequate for detailed analysis. The medico-legal implications of this revelation would be interesting, if not a matter of serious concern.

Death represents a measurable outcome of a disease process and the errors of treatment. One method of linking hospital and other medical records with the Registrar General's extract from the death certificate, in the United Kingdom, is the National Health Service Number (Acheson, 1967). It is the only identification system which approaches the criteria of being unique and universal. Possibly one reason for its absence from the identification section of most hospital medical records in the past has been its lack of availability or at least difficulty in acquiring it. Nevertheless, the assumption may have been made too readily that linkage cannot be improved using this facility. Adequate explanations to patients about where to find items such as their National Health Service Number and the reasons for fully documenting their identification details in the medical record may lead to a high level of patient collaboration (Hedley, Alexander and Innes, 1977).

Improvement in the quality and use of hospital records must be paralleled by similar improvements in their general practice counterparts. Death certification could be improved through the use of better methods of exchanging information between hospital and practice records.

Medical records and measurement of costs and effectiveness

Rising costs and demands increasingly present problems of allocating resources in the planning of health services. Options include the reduction of costs, for example by closing hospital wards and other services, or devising alternative methods of delivering care. As most of the health service costs are generated by hospitals there is increasing interest in ensuring that the services they offer are efficient and effective. Information for *ad hoc* studies on cost effectiveness and cost-benefit, for example in the treatment of benign prostatic hypertrophy has been obtained from an examination of in-patient medical records. In two such studies comparisons were made between different hospitals. The authors demonstrated the clinical, social and economic advantages of transurethral resection versus open prostatectomy (Argyrou *et al* 1974) and higher overall case-fatality rates for surgical treatment of prostatic hyperplasia in non-teaching hospitals (Ashley, Howlett, and Morris, 1971). They do not mention difficulties with the interpretation and collation of clinical information from records but the need for comparability and completeness in medical records is evident if valid comparisons are to be achieved routinely. In studying the use of scarce resources in health care, a major difficulty has been encountered in estimating the cost of treatment given to a single patient. The present system of hospital costing gives little guide to the financial implications of any change in policy or practice at ward level. One study (University of Aberdeen, 1973), specifically aimed to create a simple method of costing treatment for individual patients with different conditions and recording the use of services to allow comparisons between diseases, treatments, patients and hospitals. The team was able to use a standard method of recording drug prescriptions as a source document without modification. However, in the case of the medical record they could only concede that there was 'a vague strand of uniformity passing through the medical records'. It was difficult to retrieve information about specific items of service, many of these such as intravenous infusions, haemoglobin and ESR estimations were poorly recorded. Incoming documents, such as laboratory reports were handled so haphazardly that many might never have reached the medical record. A new method of recording investigations was developed and gained acceptance by the staff. Initially 85.8 per cent of tests were recorded at the point of ordering and confirmed by the later appearance of a report but concordance between orders and reports fell subsequently to below 80 per cent.

A review of evaluation studies in medical care reveals that, in many instances, the evaluation of the quality and costs of care is based on ascertainment of the clinical process and outcome from the content of the patient record. Attempting to achieve an objective assessment of unstructured records is a formidable task and probably of little value. Yet the design and implentation of special evaluation studies in medical care is difficult and time-consuming. The small sample size in many published reports is evidence in support of this. What is needed is the facility to extract easily and interpret with confidence the information which is accumulated through large numbers of routine patient contacts.

Medical records, record linkage, assessment of need and the prediction of risk

In a previous section, we discussed the extent to which information held in patients' records has so far been under-utilised by clinicians. However, one criticism of clinical information held by a system such as Hospital Activity Analysis is that it only provides information about events (such as hospital admissions for a particular condition) and not about the experience of individual patients. One scheme for linking information on births, deaths and discharges from hospital, in a defined population, has been operating in Oxfordshire since 1962 (Acheson, 1967). The application and use of the information has been discussed in reports on several different projects. One of these described by Acheson and Fairbairn (1973) illustrates how information from two different sources, discharges and deaths, can be utilised to determine the need for specific kinds of surveillance and monitoring and also to assess the effectiveness of programmes for screening and intervention. The study used three principal sources of data:

1. The Registrar General's Code of Operations which is included

in the patients' discharge profiles.

2. Notification of deaths amongst the defined population at risk covered by the Oxford Record Linkage Study (ORLA).

3. Estimates of the whole population in the ORLA obtained from information in the Registrar General's Decennial Census from Annual Reviews.

From this, by calculating operation rates and constructing life-tables for males and females, the proportion of survivors of an original cohort who have undergone surgical removal of an organ can be estimated for a specific point in time (e.g. each five year anniversary). Plotting the cumulative risk of organ removal for a given survivor population allows the high risk group to be described – e.g. for tonsillectomy the risk is approximately equal for the sexes and reaches its peak between 10 and 20 years; for hysterectomy the cumulative risk is 10 per cent by age 45–50 but continues to rise to 20 per cent by age 75 and for lower limb amputation the cumulative risk is 1.1 per cent at age 75 years in men and 0.2 per cent in women.

By combining information of this kind with knowledge about the pathophysiological consequences of organ removal – such as anaemia and malabsorption after partial gastrectomy or hypothyroidism and recurrent hyperthyroidism after subtotal thyroidectomy it would be possible to examine the gap between estimated *need* for aftercare and *demand* actually being made on available services. Similarly, as the authors point out, organ removal may reduce or remove the risk of certain events occurring in the future, such as cancer of the cervix following hysterectomy. Changes in the proportion of patients who are at-risk of developing diseases which are the target of screening programmes, can therefore be taken into account when assessing the effectiveness and long term outcome of this form of secondary prevention.

SUMMARY AND CONCLUSIONS

The medical record is the central focus of all our activities in the collection and utilisation of clinical information. Good quality records are essential for the delivery of care to the individual and equally for the evaluation of health services and determination of the best options in medical care.

Present methods of generating medical records in routine clinical practice have fallen behind the minimum standard necessary to meet the demands which we now make on this unique information source. A change in both methods of working and attitudes is needed if we are to progress quickly to the stage where patient records will yield uniform data which can be utilised in the measurement of services and future planning. One urgent problem concerns the interface between the clinical record and information systems, for example Hospital Activity Analysis and other procedures such as death certification. The growing demand for the development and testing of methods could be met by accepting the use of the record as a basis for audit along previously agreed guidelines, *within the context of routine practice.*

Our concepts of records, their purpose, possible future development and applications are too limited. This is particularly true in relation to their use by patients. A radical reorientation in thinking is needed by health personnel on the question of the acquisition and ownership of medical knowledge by patients and the contribution which they can make to the task of completing essential information in the record.

Our increasing knowledge about the need for therapeutic intervention, for example in chronic disease such as hypertension, highlights the problems of manpower and resources. If the known needs of defined populations are to be met in such a way that a uniformly high standard of care is provided for all – and not simply for a minority, then alternative strategies for the collection of clinical information must be developed. The delegation of many of these tasks, until now the sole responsibility of doctors, can be achieved by the design and use of explicit protocols in the form of decision-trees and checklists.

We need no reminder that health personnel are fallible in their clinical activities but the record is under-utilised as an instrument for controlling and monitoring their work. Especially when linked with automated methods of linking different types of clinical information, a logically constructed record can prevent errors in performance – a commoner source of problems than deficiencies in factual knowledge. The danger of professional obsolescence, in the face of the rapidly expanding core of clinical knowledge which must be continually assimilated after completion of basic training, has led to increasing emphasis on the need for effective methods of continuing education. The medical record can become a powerful tool in the process of continuing education and can be used as an indicator of deficiencies in clinical knowledge and the ability to apply it.

All of these issues together form an exciting challenge to health personnel and create a wealth of opportunities for the formulation and testing of new ideas in the collection and utilisation of clinical information.

ACKNOWLEDGEMENTS

I am indebted to Mrs. J. R. Beesley and Mrs. R. J. Burgass for their patience and skill in typing the manuscript. Dr. D. C. Moir, Department of Community Medicine, University of Aberdeen supplied details of the Aberdeen/Dundee drug evaluation and monitoring group.

REFERENCES

Acheson, E. D. & Fairbairn, A. S. (1973) Extent of organ removal; its importance and measurement In, *Uses of Epidemiology in Planning Health Services.* (Ed. A. M. Davies). International Epidemiological Association. Proceedings of the Sixth International Scientific Meeting. Belgrade: Savremena Administracija.

Acheson, E. D. (1967) *Medical Record Linkage.* Nuffield Provincial Hospitals Trust. Oxford University Press.

Anderson, J. & Day, J. C. (1968) New self-administered medical questionary. *British Medical Journal,* **4,** 636–638.

Argyrou, S., Blandy, J. P., Gow, J. G., Singh, M., Tresidder, G. C. & Vinnicombe, J. (1974) Price of prostatectomy. *British Medical Journal,* **3,** 511–513.

Ashbaugh, D. G. & McKean, R.,S. (1976) Continuing medical education. The philosophy and use of audit. *Journal of the American Medical Association,* **236,** 1485–1488.

Ashley, J. S. A., Howlett, A. & Morris, J. N. (1971) Case-fatality of hyperplasia of the prostate in two teaching and three regional-board hospitals, *Lancet,* **2,** 1308–1311.

Backett, E. M. & England R. (1975) How barefoot? Next steps for the medical auxiliary. *Lancet,* **2,** 1137–1141.

Barlow, D. H., Beevers, D. G., Hawthorne, V. M., Watt, H. D. & Young, G. A. R. (1977) Blood pressure measurement at screening and in general practice. *British Heart Journal,* **39,** 7–12.

Bayliss, R. I. S. & Hall, R. The Thyroid Gland. *Medicine,* **7** (second series) p. 297–320. Medical Education (International) Ltd.

Beveridge, T. & Petrie, J. C. (1972) Transfer of information about intake of drugs by patients referred to medical units. *British Medical Journal,* **2,** 37–39.

Billewicz, W. Z., Chapman, R. S., Crooks, J., Day, M. E., Gossage, J., Wayne, E. J., & Young, J. A. (1969) Statistical methods applied to the diagnosis of hypothyroidism. *Quarterly Journal of Medicine,* **38,** 255–266.

Bjorn, J. C. & Cross, H. D. (1970) *Problem Orientated Practice.* Chicago Modern Hospitals Press. McGraw-Hill Publications, Chicago.

Blackburn, H. (1973) Status and problems of the US multiple risk factor intervention trial (MRFIT). *INSERM,* **21,** 205–212.

Bodenham, K. E., & Wellman, F. (1972) *Foundations For Health Service Management.* Published for Nuffield Provincial Hospitals Trust by Oxford University Press.

Bonnar, J., Goldberg, A. & Smith, J. A. (1969) Do pregnant women take their iron? *Lancet,* **1,** 457–458.

British Medical Association Planning Unit (1969) Priorities in medicine. *British Medical Journal,* **1,** 106–108.

British Medical Association. (1970). Primary Medical Care. *British Medical Association planning unit report No. 4.*

British Medical Association. (1977) Submission of evidence to the Royal Commission on the National Health Service. *British Medical Journal,* **1,** 299–334.

Brooke, E. M. (1974). *The Current And Future use of Registers In Health Information Systems.* Offset Publication No. 8. World Health Organization.

Cahill, E. F., Etzweiler, D. D. & Freinkel, N. (1976) Editorial: 'Control' and diabetes. *New England Journal of Medicine,* **294,** 1004–1005.

Central Health Services Council (1971) *The Organisation of the Standing Advisory Committee.* HMSO.

Clayden, A. D. & Metcalfe, D. H. H. (1977) A management game for local health care planning. *The Hospital and Health Services Review*, **73**, 46–49.

Cormack, J. (1971) The general practitioner's use of medical records. *Scottish Health Service Studies No. 15.* Scottish Home and Health Department, HMSO, Edinburgh.

Crooks, J., Murray, I. P. C. & Wayne, E. J. (1959) Statistical methods applied to the clinical diagnosis of hyperthroidism. *Quarterly Journal of Medicine*, **28**, 211–234.

Crooks, J., Wayne, E. J. & Robb, R. A. (1960) A clinical method of assessing the results of therapy in thyrotoxicosis. *Lancet*, **1**, 397–401.

Crooks, J., Calder, G. & Weir, R. D. (1967) Drugs in Hospital. *Journal of the Royal College of Physicians, London*, **1**, 233–244.

Crooks, J., Clark, C. G., Caie, H. B. & Mawson, W. B. (1965) Prescribing and administration of drugs in hospital. *Lancet*, **1**, 373–378.

Crooks, J., Weir, R. D., Coull, D. C., McNab, J. W., Calder, G., Barnett, J. W. & Caie, H. B. (1967) Evaluation of a method of prescribing drugs in hospital and a new method of recording their administration. *Lancet*, **1**, 668–671.

Department of Health and Social Security, National Health Service (1969) *Hospital Activity Analysis*, (HM(69)79) London DHSS.

Department of Health and Social Security (1971) *All in a working day*. A management services (NHS) study commissioned by the Joint Working Party on the Organisation of Medical Work in hospitals. p.15 HMSO.

Department of Health and Social Security. *Notes on return form SH3: Work load.* Annual to 31st December. London DHSS.

Department of Health and Social Security and Office of Population Censuses and Surveys. *Report of Hospital In-Patient Enquiry for The Year.* Annual publication HMSO London.

Department of Health and Social Security (1977) *The Extending Role of the Clinical Nurse – Legal Implications and Training Requirements.* CMO (77)10; CNO(77)9 30th June.

Diabetic Cooperation Booklet. *Hoechst Meducation Service*, Hoechst House, Salisbury Road, Hounslow, Middlesex TW4 6JH.

Dixon, W. M., Stradling, P. & Wooton, I. D. P. (1957) Outpatient PAS therapy. *Lancet*, **2**, 871–872.

Doll, W. R. S. (1976) Monitoring of government statistics. In, *Seminars in Community Medicine, Vol. 2. Health Information and Monitoring.* (Editors R. M. Acheson, D. Hall, L. Aird) Oxford University Press.

Dollery, C. T., Beilin, L. J., Bulpitt, C. J., Coles, E. C., Johnson, B. F., Munro-Faure, A. D. & Turner, S. C. (1977). Initial care of hypertensive patients: Influence of different types of clinical records. *British Heart Journal*, **39**, 181–185.

Ennals, D. (1977) *The Times*, 29th January.

Essex, B. J. (1976) *Diagnostic Pathways in Clinical Medicine.* Edinburgh: Churchill Livingstone. Longman Group Ltd.

Fairbairn, A. S., Wood, C. H. & Fletcher, C. M. (1959) Variability in answers to a questionnaire on respiratory symptoms. *British Journal of Preventive and Social Medicine*, **14**, 175–189.

Feinstein, A. R. (1967) *Clinical Judgement.* Baltimore: William and Wilkins.

Fendall, N. R. E. (1972) *Auxiliaries in Health Care: Programs in Developing Countries.* Baltimore.

Gumpel, J. M. & Mason, A. M. S. (1974) Self-administered clinical questionnaire for out-patients. *British Medical Journal*, **2**, 209–212.

Gurney, C., Owen, S. G., Hall, R., Roth, M., Harper, M. & Smart, G. A. (1970) Newcastle thyrotoxicosis index. *Lancet*, **2**, 1275–1278.

Hall, G. H. (1972) Experiences with out-patient medical questionnaires. *British*

Medical Journal, **1**, 42-45.

Hall, M. R. P. (1974) Geriatric medicine and its role in the care of the elderly. *Medicine*, **25**, pp. 1465-1480. Medical Education (International) Ltd.

Hart, J. T. (1970) Semi-continuous screening of a whole community for hypertension. *Lancet*, **2**, 223-226.

Heasman, M. A. & Lipworth, L. (1966) *Accuracy Of Certification Of Causes Of Death*. General Register Office, Studies on medical and population subjects. No. 2. HMSO.

Heasman, M. A. (1968) Scottish hospital in-patient statistics - sources and uses. *Health Bulletin*, **4**, 10-18.

Heasman, M. A. & Carstairs, V. (1971) Inpatient management: variations in some aspects of practice in Scotland. *British Medical Journal*, **1**, 495-498.

Heasman, M. A. (1976) SCRIPS: Success or failure. In, *A Question of Quality: Roads to Assurance In Medical Care*. (Edited by G. McLachlan) pp. 173-185. Published for Nuffield Provincial Hospitals Trust by Oxford University Press.

Hedley, A. J. (1977) Computerized Central Registers. In *Medico-Social Management of Inherited Metabolic Disease* Ed. D. N. Raine, Medical and Technical Publishing Ltd.

Hedley, A. J., Alexander, E. & Innes, G. (1977) Patient identification and documentation of causes of death in a follow-up register. *Health Bulletin*, March, 73-78.

Hedley, A. J. & Ryan, M. P. (1978) Problem oriented records and anticipatory care for the elderly, *in preparation*.

Heller, R. F. & Rose, G. A. (1977a) Current management of hypertension in hospital. *British Medical Journal*, **1**, 1441-1442.

Heller, R. F. & Rose, G. A. (1977b) Current management of hypertension in general practice. *British Medical Journal*, **1**, 1442-1444.

Hill, R. D. (1976) Running a diabetic clinic. *British Journal of Hospital Medicine*, **16**, 218-226.

Hodgkins, E. (1965) Listen: The patient. *New England Journal of Medicine*, **274**, 657-661.

Horrocks, J. C. & de Dombal, F. T. (1975) Diagnosis of dyspepsia from data collected by a physician's assistant. *British Medical Journal*, **3**, 421-423.

Horrocks, J. C., Lambert, D. E., McAdam, W. A. F., Morgan, A. C., Pacsoo, C., Darnborough, A. & de Dombal, F. T. (1976). Transfer of computer-aided diagnosis from one geographical area to another. *Gut*, **17**, 640-644.

Joint National Committee on Detection, Evaluation and Treatment of High Blood Pressure (1977) A co-operative study. *Journal of the American Medical Association*, **237**, 255-261.

Joyce, C. R. B. (1962) Patient co-operation and the sensitivity of clinical trials. *Journal of Chronic Diseases*, **15**, 1025-1036.

Judd, S. L., O'Leary, E., Read, P. & Fox, C. (1976) The changing role of nurses in the management of diabetes. *British Journal of Hospital Medicine*, **16**, 251-255.

Kannel, W. B. & Dawber, T. R. (1974) Hypertension as an ingredient of a cardiovascular risk profile. *British Journal of Hospital Medicine*, **11**, 508-523.

Koran, L. (1975) The reliability of clinical methods, data and judgements. *New England Journal of Medicine*, **293**, 642-646 and 695-701.

Lefever, R., West, J. & Trevelyan, T. (1977) *Self-administered questionnaire for new patients in general practice*.

Leading Article (1966) Accuracy of death certificates. *Lancet*, **2**, 1349.

Macdonald, C. J. (1976) Protocol-based computer reminders, the quality of care and the non-perfectability of man. *New England Journal of Medicine*, **295**, 1351-1355.

McIntyre, N. (1974) Obtaining information from medical records. *Journal of The Royal College of Physicians, London*, **8**, 267-275.

Mahler, H. (1974) in *The Medical Assistant: An Intermediate Level Of Health Care Personnel* (Edited by Pitcairn, D. M., and Flahault, D.) Public Health Paper,

No. 60, World Health Organisation.

Medical Research Council (1966) *Questionnaire on respiratory symptoms.*

Ministry of Health (1968) *First Report Of The Joint Working Party On The Organisation Of Medical Work In Hospitals* (Cogwheel Report) London, HMSO.

Ministry of Health (1959) *Hospital O & M Service Report No. 2.* Medical records and secretarial services. HMSO.

Morley, D. (1973) *Paediatric Priorities In The Developing World.* London: Butterworths.

Morris, D., Buckler, M., Goss, F., Harvie, J., Williams, R. & Willox, I. (1974) *Cogstats: Some Notes On The Use Of Statistics In The Divisional Management Of Hospital Medical Services.* King Edward's Hospital Fund for London.

Murray, F. A. & Topley, L. (1974) Patients as record holders. *Health and Social Service Journal,* July 27, 1675.

O'Grady, F. W., Lambert, H. P. & Begent, R. H. J. (1975) Sensible prescribing: V. Diarrhoea and vomiting. **Practitioner,* **214,** 661–665.

Porter, A. M. W. (1969) Drug defaulting in general practice. *British Medical Journal,* **1,** 218–222.

Rang, E. H., Acheson, E. D. & O'Connor, B. T. (1968) Clinical significance of deaths after discharge from hospital unrecorded in the hospital notes. *Lancet,* **2,** 908–910.

Reports of the Committee on Nursing (1972) (Chairman: Prof. A. Briggs), *Cmnd 5115* London: HMSO.

Report of Medical Research Council Working Party on Mild to Moderate Hypertension (1977) Randomised controlled trial of treatment for mild hypertension: design and pilot trial. *British Medical Journal,* **1,** 1437–1440.

Ritchie, D. M., Boyle, J. A., McInnes, J. M., Janani, M. K., Dalakos, T. G., Grieveson, P. & Buchanan, W. W. (1968) Clinical studies with an articular index for the assessment of joint tenderness in patients with rheumatoid arthritis. *Quarterly Journal of Medicine,* **37,** 393–406.

Robinson, D. W., Walmsley, G. L., Horrocks, J. C., Milson, P., Jenkins, D. M., de Dombal, F. T. & Scott, J. S. (1975) Histories obtained by two stage questionnaire with automated transcript in specialist gynaecological practice. *British Medical Journal,* **4,** 510–513.

Rose, G. A. & Blackburn, H. (1968) *Cardiovascular survey methods.* World Health Organisation.

Rosenow, C. E. Jr. (1971) Medical knowledge self-assessment programmes. Paper presented at the 173rd Annual Meeting of the Medical Chirurgical Faculty of the State of Maryland, Baltimore. April 1971. Cited by Dubin, S. S. (1972) Obsolescence of lifelong education: a choice for the profession. *American Journal of Psychology,* **4,** 510–513.

Rowe, R. G. & Brewer, W. (1972) *Hospital Activity Analysis.* Computers in Medicine Series. (General Ed. Hill D. W.). London: Butterworths.

Royal College of General Practitioners. (1973) Present state and future needs of general practice (3rd edition) *Report from General Practice No. 16.*

Scottish Home and Health Department (1967) *Organisation Of Medical Work In The Hospital Service In Scotland.* Edinburgh, HMSO.

Scottish Hospital In-Patient Statistics. (1961–68) (1964–70) *Scottish Home and Health Department and Scottish Health Statistics,* 1969– Annual Publication. Edinburgh, HMSO.

Seidl, L. G., Thornton, G. F., Smith, J. W. & Cluff, L. E. (1966) Studies on the epidemiology of adverse drug reactions: III. Reactions in patients on a general medical service. *Bulletin of the Johns Hopkins Hospital,* **119,** 299–315.

Sheldon, M. G. (1976) Patient-filled questionnaires. *Update,* October, 651–660.

Small, W. P. (1966) Living records. *Lancet,* **1,** 1146–1147.

---

* See also Practitioner issue numbers 1284, 1285, 1281, 1289 of volume 214 for algorithms on osteoarthrosis, otitis media, urinary tract infection and epilepsy.

Smart, G. A. (1975) Monitoring in medicine. *Journal of the Royal College of Physicians, London*, **9**, 355–70.

Smith, A. J. (1975) Sensible prescribing; IX. Management of hypertension. *Practitioner*, **215**, 327–334.

Society of Actuaries (1959) *Build and blood pressure study*. 1 and 2. Chicago.

Sox, H. C., Sox, C. H. & Tompkins, R. K. (1973) The training of physicians assistants: Use of a clinical algorithm system for patient care, audit of performance and education. *New England Journal of Medicine*, **288**, 818–824.

Spitzer, W. O., Sackett, D. L., Sibley, J. C., Roberts, R. S., Gent, M., Kergin, D. J., Hackett, B. C. & Olynich, A. (1974) The Burlington randomised trial of the nurse practitioner. *New England Journal of Medicine*, **290**, 251–256.

Tait, I. & Stevens, J. (1973) The problem-orientated medical record in general practice. *Journal of the Royal College of General Practitioners*, **23**, 311–315.

Tulloch, A. J., Fowler, G. H., McMullan, J. J. & Spence, J. M. (1975) Hospital discharge reports: content and design. *British Medical Journal*, **4**, 443–446.

University of Aberdeen (1973) *Patient Costing Study*. (Editors Russell, E. M., Dingwall-Fordyce, I. & Harper, D. R.). University of Aberdeen.

Vignos, P. J., Parker, W. T. & Thompson, H. M. (1976) Evaluation of a clinic education program for patients with rheumatoid arthritis. *Journal of Rheumatology*, **3**, (part 2) 155–165.

Weed, L. L. (1973) Problem oriented medical records: can it work in general practice? Audio-tape 73/10. *Medical Recording Service Foundation*. Royal College of General Practitioners.

Wheatley, D. M. & Unwin, A. W. (1972) *The Algorithm Writers Guide*. London: Longman Group.

Weiner, S. & Nathanson, M. (1976) Physical examination: frequently observed errors. *Journal of the American Medical Association*, **236**, 852–855.

Willcox, D. R. C., Gillan, R. & Hare, E. H. (1965) Do psychiatric outpatients take their drugs? *British Medical Journal*, **2**, 790–792.

Williamson, J., Stoke, I. H., Gray, S., Fisher, M., Smith, A., McGhee, A. & Stephenson, E. (1964) Old people at home: their unreported needs. *Lancet*, **1**, 1117–1120.

Wilson, G. (1976) The Hospital Health Services Research Unit in the University Department of Medicine, Western Infirmary, Glasgow. In, *A Question of Quality: Roads To Assurance In Medical Care* (Edited by McLachlan, G.) Published for Nuffield Provincial Hospitals Trust by Oxford University Press.

World Health Organisation (1967) *International Classification of Diseases*. Eighth Revision. **1**, 121–122. Geneva. World Health Organisation.

2

The principles of the problem orientated medical record

NEIL McINTYRE

Reader, Academic Department of Medicine, Royal Free Hospital, Pond Street, London; Clinical Sub-Dean, Royal Free Hospital School of Medicine

INTRODUCTION

For this you keep a lab notebook. Everything gets written down, formally, so that you know at all times where you are, where you've been, where you're going and where you want to get. In scientific work and electronics technology this is necessary because otherwise the problems get so complex you get lost in them and confused and forget what you know and what you don't know and have to give up. In cycle maintenance things are not that involved, but when confusion starts it's a good idea to hold it down by making everything formal and exact. Sometimes just the act of writing down the problems straightens out your head as to what they really are.

The logical statements entered into the notebook are broken down into six categories: (1) statement of the problem, (2) hypotheses as to the cause of the problem, (3) experiments designed to test each hypothesis, (4) predicted results of the experiments, (5) observed results of the experiments and (6) conclusions from the results of the experiments. This is not different from the formal arrangement of many college and high-school lab notebooks but the purpose here is no longer just busywork. The purpose now is precise guidance of thoughts that will fail if they are not accurate.
The Art of Motor Cycle Maintenance   *Robert Pirsig (1974)*

A patient's case notes are very important. They record symptoms and signs and the results of past investigations; they remind us about drugs prescribed on previous occasions and about tests for which results are awaited; they describe past illnesses, important risk factors, and indicate social and psychological factors which might influence our management of the patient. As medical care becomes more complex our records become more valuable to us; this is evident from the dismay, distress or anger which we exhibit when we have to see a patient whose notes are missing.

Records are not just *aides-memoire* for individual doctors. Many doctors may be involved in the care of a single patient. If their efforts are not coordinated care will be less efficient, may be ineffective, and occasionally will be dangerous. Medical records should help doctors to communicate and so improve the continuity of care.

One might imagine that we as doctors would take pains over our records so that we could find important data quickly and easily. We rarely do. The general standard is appalling, both in hospitals and in general practice. The content of records is usually inadequate and their structure chaotic. It may be impossible to find required information at all, let alone quickly and easily. Entries may be uninterpretable and sometimes we cannot even understand our own notes.

Why are they so bad? Mainly because of apathy. We acknowledge the deficiencies of our own records, and complain about those of others, but few try to improve them. Some may be daunted by the size of the problem; it is no easy matter to bring order out of the present chaos, and there are no material incentives to encourage those who might be willing to try. Others might be worried that colleagues would resist change. Doctors are individuals. Accustomed to 'clinical freedom' we are not renowned for our willingness to collaborate over such matters and there may be genuine concern whether a record system designed by others would be suitable for our own needs. The would-be reformer might be justifiably pessimistic about the prospects of success. He might even find if difficult to bring doctors together to discuss medical records; many are apathetic about the subject and most doctors, busy and overcommitted, are tired of meetings of any kind.

Another reason for the poor quality of medical records is their neglect during clinical training. As undergraduates we have all been taught how to record, as well as collect, a 'history and physical examination'. Most medical schools use a similar format which has much to recommend it. But it is taught as an idealised format and students soon discover that teachers, when writing their own case notes, do not practise what they preach. The reasons for 'modifications' are not made clear to students and when, due to pressure of work, they find the 'ideal' version unsatisfactory they, like their teachers, discard it. Without a suitable alternative their records deteriorate and become chaotic.

Although they may have some idea about recording a history and physical examination few students have any idea how to record management plans or useful notes on the progress of the patient. These areas are virtually ignored in medical school and the consequences are evident whenever one refers to clinical records.

Students recognise the importance of medical records and believe that more instruction should be given on writing and using them (Hughes, Lloyd and McIntyre, 1978). They expect to write up the history and physical examination but complain that their teachers pay little attention to these efforts and that they are disinterested about the recording of progress notes. Students find it valuable both to write clinical casenotes and to discuss them with teachers; it is a pity that so few teachers use them for educational purposes (*See* Ch. 5).

Our neglect of records in medical schools has two important consequences. Teachers' attitudes are transmitted to students; this might explain, or contribute to, the apathy of graduates towards medical records. Secondly because students do not study medical records, or the general problems of communication, they are unable subsequently to plan a record system appropriate to their needs.

There have been official attempts to improve the standards of records in hospitals and in general practice. 'Unit filing' has been adopted in most British hospitals. This means that notes on one patient, although originating in different departments, are now kept together in one file (with occasional exceptions for psychiatric and venereology records). This simple change has been helpful. In the Tunbridge (1965) and Walker (1967, 1973) reports excellent recommendations were made about the design of clinical documents for use in National Health Service hospitals. But the inclusion of 'standardisation' in the titles of these reports antagonised many consultants who feared restriction of their 'right' to keep records as they wished. This was unfortunate but if a medical record system is to be created which will meet today's requirements collaboration is essential and a certain amount of standardisation is inevitable.

There have also been attempts to improve general practice records and several changes have been suggested (Curtis, 1976). These have not gained widespread acceptance and most records have changed little over the years. Currently there is pressure to change general practice records from the present size (7 in. × 4½ in.) to international A4, and so bring them into line with hospital and other health care records. Unfortunately a change in the size of the records will not guarantee improved quality.

THE PRINCIPLES OF DESIGN OF GOOD MEDICAL RECORDS

Certain requirements must be satisfied in the design of a medical record system.

Records must be available when they are needed. Missing records are useless no matter how well they are written. Computers can solve the problems of availability (*See* Ch. 6) but until they are in common use for storing medical records we must rely on manual systems and should try to improve their efficiency.

Medical records must be easy to understand. They must be legible and written in a language with which the reader is familiar. For this reason jargon and unusual abbreviations should be avoided.

The information within a record should be correct and entered in context. It should be adequate, at least for the purposes of those who usually use the record.

We should be able to find information quickly. It is easier to do so if records have a standard structure with which all users are familiar and if key points are emphasised by larger writing, by underlining or by the use of colours. Information is also retrieved more easily if the record is kept as small as possible, by avoiding unnecessary entries and by the use of flow charts for laboratory results or for certain clinical observations.

A good medical record system would have other useful characteristics. It would simplify classification and coding by trained clerical staff and facilitate the extraction of data for planning or for clinical research. It might guide the collection of clinical information by including check lists or by leaving spaces for routinely collected data. Its records would be presented in such a way that the logic of clinical activity is preserved allowing us to use the record to evaluate the quality of the care provided.

A new medical record system should be compatible with eventual computerisation. The potential benefits of computerisation are obvious – immediate access, record linkage between hospitals and with general practitioners, and rapid availability of data for research and for health care planning. Important reference material on drugs and diseases etc. can also be made instantly available. Effective computerisation may seem a far cry from the poor quality records of today, but an outstanding system has already been developed (*See* Ch. 6).

PROBLEM ORIENTATED MEDICAL RECORDS (POMR*)

One system satisfies many of the principles outlined above. This is the

---

*The abbreviation POMR will be used for both singular (. . . record) and plural (. . . records) forms of the title.

Problem Orientated System of medical records, introduced by Lawrence Weed (1969). A Problem Orientated Medical Record is made up of four main parts:

1. A problem list
2. A defined data base
3. Plans   } titled and numbered with
4. Progress notes } respect to problems

The problem list

The problem list is the key to POMR. It is a list of the clinically significant events in a patient's life and highlights the factors which might affect management. It should appear on the cover or front page of the notes and act as an index or table of contents (Figs 2.1a and 2.1b). This list is known as the 'permanent' problem list.

A problem list should contain *all* problems, and include established diagnoses, pathophysiological states (such as cardiac or respiratory failure) and symptoms, abnormal physical signs and laboratory investigations which are potentially important but not encompassed by a disease or syndrome already in the list. Other important factors influencing patient care, such as psychiatric problems, social problems, risk factors and past illnesses should also be included.

An entry into the problem list should be endorsed with the date of the initial plan for that problem, or the date of the first note about it. If the record is kept chronologically we can then follow the problem easily from the beginning (*See* problems 1 and 2 in Figs 2.1a, 2.5 and 2.7). The date column should not be used to record when the patient first recognised the problem, or when it was noted in other sets of records: if it is necessary to record such information then it can be included in the title of the problem e.g. 'epigastric pain since 1953'; 'myocardial infarction, (St. Swithin's Hospital) 1967'.

It is important that items in a problem list should, as far as possible, be statements of fact at the level of understanding of the writer. The recording of guesses obscures the true problem and may even prevent correct diagnosis. Entries such as:

Diagnosis: ? duodenal ulcer
             ? cholecystitis
             ? pancreatitis

are common in conventional records but represent a loss of information rather than a gain. They should not be found in a problem list – instead one should state the true problem; in this example it would have been 'upper abdominal pain'. The diagnostic level at which problems can be stated will depend on available information

PROBLEM LIST	Hospital No. Surname OTHER M/F First Names A.N. M/S/W Fig 2.1a D. of B. 1922

PROBLEM NUMBER	I.C.D. No.	ACTIVE PROBLEMS Include Symptoms, Signs and Abnormal Investigations not Explained by Another Entry. Social and Psychiatric Problems Should Also Be Included.	DATE ENTERED	INACTIVE PROBLEMS Include Major Past Illness, Operations or Hypersensitivities. Do Not Include Problems for Which You Will Provide Active Care.
1		CHRONIC LIVER DISEASE	5.10.73	
2		THROMBOCYTOPENIA	5.10.73	
3		CIGARETTE SMOKER – HEAVY	5.10.73	
4		OBESITY	5.10.73	
5			3.1.76 ←	URINARY INFECTION – 1968
6				PULMONARY TB – 1950
7				DUODENAL ULCER – 1960
8				PENICILLIN HYPERSENSITIVITY
9		EPIDIDYMO–ORCHITIS	3.1.76	
10		URETHRAL STRICTURE	17.4.76	
11				
12				
13				
14				
15				

RF 684

Figs. 2.1a and b Examples of Problem Lists. For details see text.

and on the knowledge and experience with which the doctor can interpret it.

If new data help to establish a diagnosis, or lead to a more precise definition of a problem, the problem list can be amended; the original entry should not be erased but linked by an arrow to the new entry which retains the original number (e.g. problem 1, Fig. 2.1b). If the

PROBLEM LIST			Hospital No.	M/F
			Surname PATEL	
			First Names A.	M/S/W
Fig 2.1b			D. of B. 1946	

PROBLEM NUMBER	I.C.D. No.	ACTIVE PROBLEMS Include Symptoms, Signs and Abnormal Investigations not Explained by Another Entry. Social and Psychiatric Problems Should Also Be Included.	DATE ENTERED	INACTIVE PROBLEMS Include Major Past Illness, Operations or Hypersensitivities. Do Not Include Problems for Which You Will Provide Active Care.
1		R AXILLARY LYMPHADENOPATHY	18.10.71	
		→ TUBERCULOSIS	29.10.71 →	
2		FEVER → # 1	18.10.71 29.10.71	
3		LOSS OF WEIGHT → # 1	18.10.71 29.10.71	
4		DOESN'T READ ENGLISH	18.10.71	
5				SENSITIVITY TO INAH
6		DOMESTIC/FINANCIAL PROBLEMS	5.5.72	
7		IRON DEFICIENCY ANAEMIA	20.12.72 →	
8				
9				
10				
11				
12				
13				
14				
15				

RF 684

date of the amendment is recorded it is a simple matter, by referring to the notes for that day, to review the evidence for the change of title. When several items of the problem list prove to be explicable by one condition this should be entered in place of the first item and should take its number: the other items should be struck out and their numbers should not be used again (Fig. 2.1b Nos 2 & 3). When new problems arise they are added to the list. Thus the problem list is not a static record but becomes a dynamic statement of the patient's illness which allows a rapid assessment of the situation at any given moment.

Occasionally one disease has several manifestations; e.g. a patient with cirrhosis of the liver may suffer from jaundice, ankle oedema, ascites, portal-systemic encephalopathy and bleeding from oesophageal varices. If the complications are minor and require no special investigations or therapy, they can be left out of the problem list; alternatively they can be included in the statement of the main problem, e.g.

1. Cirrhosis of the liver – with jaundice.

If complications require individual management they can be listed as separate problems e.g.

1. Cirrhosis of the liver
2. Ascites – 2° to problem 1

```
R M    Male    Age 53

10.10.76  2    ASCITES

               S  Abdomen more comfortable.  Ankles no longer swollen.

               O  Girth 90 cm (from 96).  Weight down to 63.4 kg

               A  Good response - see flow chart.

               P  Rx - Frusemide → 40 mg

                      Spironolactone → 100 mg qds.

          3    PORTAL SYSTEMIC ENCEPHALOPATHY

               O  Memory now good.  Well orientated.  No flap.

               A  Improved ++

               P  Mx - Repeat EEG - ?  Back to normal.

                      Rx - Relax protein restriction → 80 g

          4    BLEEDING VARICES

               O  BP 90/50 at 9 a.m.  Now melaena.  Given 2 units blood.
                  BP now stable 130/80.
               P  Wait and see.

          3    PSE

               O  Slight flap.

               P  Mx - Postpone EEG.

                      Rx - Mag sulph enema

                           Increase lactulose

                           Protein to 20 g again.
```

Fig. 2.2 An example of progress notes in which the individual problems are complications of the same disease, the title of which was listed as Problem 1, Cirrhosis.

3. Portal-systemic encephalopathy – 2° to problem 1
4. Bleeding oesophageal varices – 2° to problem 1

The course of each can then be followed separately in the notes as in Figure 2.2.

The problem list is formulated following review of the data base. Problems which require action are called 'active' problems. Others may require no immediate action for the purposes of diagnosis, monitoring, treatment, or patient education. It may still be advisable to display them on the problem list because knowledge of their existence may affect the management of other problems. For example a history of treated tuberculosis or of a previous duodenal ulcer would weigh against the use of steroids, and known hypersensitivity to a drug would clearly restrict its use. Weed (1969) advocates that such conditions should be listed separately in the problem list under the heading 'inactive problems'. An active problem may become inactive and vice versa. Such change of status should be recorded with an arrow and should be dated (e.g. Fig. 2.1b, problems 1 and 7); again the presence of the date allows the evidence for change in status to be found in the record.

Some problems can be entered immediately into the problem list, particularly in the 'inactive' column (e.g. myocardial infarct in 1965, penicillin hypersensitivity). Other entries may profitably be delayed. One should avoid listing items in the permanent problem list if they are likely to be deleted or altered within a short period of time: clinical features may be puzzling when a patient first presents but easy to explain when the results of appropriate investigations are available. For this reason Weed suggested that 24 hours might be allowed before making entries in the *permanent* problem list. His choice of time was arbitrary and it may be convenient to delay for a longer period. The delay should not be too long as the possession of the problem list confers a number of important benefits.

Until the permanent problem list is prepared we can use the headings of 'initial plans' to serve as a reminder about active problems or we can construct a supplementary problem list. This may be useful even when a permanent problem list is available. It can be used to record temporary or self-limiting conditions; these can be transferred to the permanent list if they become more serious or if they occur with unusual frequency. It can also be used as a rough sheet on which any member of the health care team can suggest problem headings, or on which vague problems can remain prior to their resolution or to their elucidation and transfer to the permanent list (Fig. 3.7).

The permanent problem list should be constructed and updated by the medical personnel in charge of the patient. Updating should be done promptly. The problem list allows us to choose the problems for attention during a consultation. Therefore the list should be complete. We might miss something important if we acted on the basis of an out of date problem list (but even that is usually preferable to the absence of a problem list!)

The data base

Before we can formulate a comprehensive list of problems we must review what we have learned about the patient. In the Problem Orientated system this information is called the DATA BASE. Many doctors, especially in Britain, dislike the term considering it as jargon – unattractive and unnecessary; but it is now widely used and no better alternative has been proposed.

There is a good deal of misunderstanding about Weed's concept of a data base. Critics of POMR attack the data base as a rigid concept leading to excessive data collection. They object to Weed's insistence that data which are to be collected routinely should be clearly defined, and claim that doctors cannot routinely collect the large data base which he advocates. *But Weed's approach is really very flexible.*

The information contained in the data base is of two types. *Problem specific information* relates to the complaints or problems with which the patient presented, or which were elicited during history taking. In an emergency or when time is short problem specific information may be all that is collected, but for obvious reasons such limitation of data collection is potentially hazardous; most doctors therefore collect some *routine information* – to familiarise themselves with previously recognised disorders, to detect unsuspected conditions and to learn about social problems or risk factors. This routine information constitutes Weed's *defined data base.*

This '*defined* data base' is the information which a doctor, or group of doctors, considers necessary to care properly for his patients. Its size should be such that, under usual conditions, complete collection is possible for all patients. The content and size of this defined data base should be determined by the type of patient seen, and by the time and resources available to the doctor, or group of doctors, concerned. Completion of Weed's own large defined data base (Weed, 1969, 1974) depends on the use of ancillary methods of collection; it was designed to provide large amounts of information, but it was not intended that doctors should have to collect it all.

Critics also complain that the recording of clinical information is constrained by the structure of the Problem Orientated data base. *But the choice of format is not crucial.* The complete data base (problem specific and defined) is analogous to a conventional 'history and physical examination' and can be written out in the same way. It should contain the information needed for efficient and effective patient care. This can be gleaned from several sources; from the history, which will be obtained from the patient, or from relatives, friends or old notes; from physical examination; or from laboratory investigations.

The complete data base, like the conventional 'history and physical examination', might include the presenting complaint(s), an account of the history of the present illness, and a systems review, past history, family history, psycho-social history and drug history, as well as a description of the findings on physical examination. It should also include the results of routine laboratory and ward tests. Weed argues for the inclusion of a *patient profile*, which describes an average working day and a typical day of leisure; this helps to indicate the effect of illness on daily activities, and *vice versa*, and allows us to adjust our management to the particular requirements of each patient.

The main component of the 'history of the presenting illness' must be the description of the presenting complaint(s). This should reflect a systematic approach to the collection of data. If the patient had a pain then the description should tell us where it was; its character and severity; how long it lasted, how it started and stopped, and for what periods the patient was free of pain; it should indicate what made the pain better or worse, and what features were associated with the pain in one way or another. Other symptoms such as cough or breathlessness can be described similarly.

The 'history of the presenting illness' will often go beyond the bounds of a single system, such as the cardiovascular or nervous systems, not only because there may be several presenting complaints but also because we may actively search for associated symptoms in other systems. It should, ideally, include an elaboration of all of the positive responses obtained on systems review. This is rarely practical as there are usually too many positives for even a brief description of all of them. We must try to judge which of them deserve elaboration.

When there are several different complaints each may be dealt with separately in the 'history of the presenting illness' and this usually allows the clearest presentation (Fig. 2.3a). Occasionally the patient's story is too confusing for clear separation of the individual problems; a chronological account may then be the only practical way to tell the story (Fig. 2.3b).

Conventionally we write up a new 'history and physical examination' whenever a patient is readmitted to hospital. Much of it, such as past history, family history and social history, need only be recorded once, if the initial version is accurate, complete and can be found easily

J C   Male   Age 65

Retired Company Accountant

31.10.75   HISTORY OF PRESENT ILLNESS

        Atrial Fibrillation

                Heart 'jumped' for 5 mins while carrying heavy
                parcel on 20 June. Happened again 3 weeks later.
                ECG by GP showed atrial fibrillation. Was given
                Digoxin 0.25 mg bd. Palpitations have occurred
                for about 5 mins three times weekly ever since.
                Don't really trouble him.

        Diarrhoea, Loss of Weight

                Diarrhoea began suddenly on 12 September. 4-6 stools
                daily since then. Originally pale, not offensive,
                flushed easily. No blood or mucus. GP attributed
                it to Digoxin which was stopped but there was no
                improvement. Three weeks later the stools were
                bulky, 'oily' and wouldn't flush. Weight loss of
                1 stone despite good appetite. Stool cultures were
                negative. Little relief with Mist Kaolin or Morph.
                No other gastrointestinal symptoms.

        Depression

                Gradual onset of depression over last year or so.
                Unhappy about his recent retirement and a number of
                family problems. Feels lethargic and has lost
                interest in most of his usual activities. Wakes
                early and finds it difficult to face the day. Can't
                concentrate and finds it difficult to make decisions.
                Cries occasionally and has thought of suicide.
                Diazepam doesn't help. Started amitryptiline but
                they didn't help and he stopped taking them after a
                week or so.

Fig. 2.3a An example of a history in which the main complaints were best dealt with separately. The patient presented with three clearly defined problems and an excellent letter from the G.P. It was therefore easy to write a history for each symptom. It transpired that the fibrillation was due to thyrotoxicosis which also contributed to the diarrhoea – but in addition he had chronic pancreatitis which needed treatment!

in the notes. It would seem sensible to store this information in a special section of the notes; we should check its accuracy occasionally and amend it when necessary. Information obtained by systems review can also be stored economically and efficiently in a special section of the record (Fig. 2.10b).

Great efforts should be made to avoid the recording of redundant information. An adequate account written by one doctor should not be duplicated. Others should confirm its accuracy by checking with the patient or with other sources of information and additions and corrections should be made only if they are necessary.

The routine part of the data base should contain the answers to questions which are asked routinely, regardless of the nature of the presenting complaint(s). Ideally it would contain all the information which might conceivably affect the management of the patient. In practice, of course, it is impossible to collect such a large amount of data and we must decide what information we really do need.

Some information is obviously vital e.g. about penicillin hypersensitivity or bleeding disorders. We must know if the patient smokes or drinks excessively or if he has asymptomatic hypertension or chronic bronchitis. We should also seek information which might otherwise be withheld from us. Many patients are embarrassed about problems such as stress incontinence, impotence or marital difficulties and may not disclose them voluntarily even though they may be happy to do so once the subject has been broached; information may also be withheld because of a lapse of memory or because the patient does not realise its importance.

The number of possible questions is clearly very large and we must think very carefully about those which will be asked routinely. We

```
M T  Male  Age 29

17.1.77   PC Epigastric Discomfort

     HPI

     From Dominica.  Here 19 years.   Works on electric
     wiring.   Keen games player.   Perfectly fit and well
     until 1971 - began to get pains in the right loin and
     over the bladder.   Went with micturition.  Continued
     until about 18 months ago when had a complete check up
     at another hospital.   A small duodenal ulcer was found
     but was told nothing wrong with the kidneys.   Was
     treated with alkalies and had no pain for 6 months.
     About a year ago noticed fluttering on the right side
     of the epigastrium and over the praecordium.   His GP
     said it was 'nerves' and gave him tablets.   This
     fluttering around the heart has persisted ever since.
     It is not a pain - just a 'jump'.   It may occur 4 times
     in ½ hour - then goes away.   Doesn't occur every day,
     but may come every day for a month and then stops for
     a month.

     Also has had fleeting pains for last 2 years - which
     last a second or so - all over chest and abdomen.  Has
     pains in ankle joints but only after walking for long
     distances.  Is losing hair more rapidly than he should.
     Admits to depression because his girl friend doesn't
     always do as he wants her to and this makes it difficult
     for him to relax.   Is tired on rising, has panicky
     feelings, is lethargic and finds it difficult to
     concentrate.
```

Fig. 2.3b This history is far from ideal. It would have been difficult to deal with individual problems separately because it quickly became apparent that his symptoms were quite various and were not due to a duodenal ulcer as suggested by his general practitioner.

must decide how we would use the answers as this should determine the priority to be given to their collection.

Our *defined* data base should not be '*fixed*' on completion. If there are important omissions we should incorporate them subsequently, and should delete items which prove useless.

Definition and standardisation of a data base help to ensure complete collection. Missing answers are noticed more easily and can be filled in later. A data base does not have to be completed during one consultation; it can be built up over a period of time. This blunts the criticism that complete collection is impossible if the defined data base is a large one.

In an emergency it is obviously inappropriate to set about collecting a large routine data base. The patient with pulmonary oedema, coma or respiratory failure has to be treated even if we are not in possession of all the facts. The data base can be completed subsequently when the patient improves or when old notes become available. When we are unable to collect important data we may decide that the first entry in the problem list should be *incomplete data base*; this would remind us to collect the missing information at a later stage. Data collection should always be considered as an on-going process and inaccuracies corrected whenever they are found.

```
F P Male   Age 59

1.12.69

        Impression:     Acute on chronic Bronchitis

                        ?  LV failure

                        ?  Pulmonary embolism - but no obvious cause

                        Myocardial ischaemia

                        Gout

                        Fistula in Ano    ? Crohn's

Investigations                  Rx

ECG                             IV Aminophylline - 250mg

Chest X-ray                     IV Lasix - 20 mg

Full blood count                Lasix tabs

Urea and electrolytes           K⁺ supplements

Sputum-culture                  Bronchodilators

Cytoscopy                       Antibiotics - after sputum culture

MSU                             Probenecid

Pulmonary function tests

Enzymes

LFTs - electrophoresis
```

Fig. 2.4 This unedited list of diagnosis, investigations and therapy is better than those usually found in conventional notes. It does not mention hepatosplenomegaly although it was noted in the physical examination (and may have been the reason for ordering liver function tests!) An extensor plantar had also been found. It would have been simple to specify what potassium supplements and bronchodilators were prescribed.

Emergencies highlight the value of the problem list and of the defined data base. In a crisis the doctor, and more importantly the patient, benefits greatly from a list of previously recognised problems and from easy access to information collected at an earlier time. Conventional records are often unhelpful in times of crisis.

Initial plans
In conventional hospital notes the record of the history and physical examination is followed by a statement of the most likely diagnosis, or by a short list of possible diagnoses (Fig. 2.4). The statement of provisional diagnoses in this form has at least two practical disadvantages. First, interest is focussed only on the 'main' features in the clinical history; findings that are not clearly related to the provisional diagnoses may be ignored even though they deserve attention. Second if only one 'diagnosis' is recorded it may be retained as a label even if it is unconfirmed; this stifles diagnostic activity. After the provisional diagnoses we may find a list of the investigations requested and less commonly a list of the drugs prescribed (Fig. 2.4). The doctor may have had several purposes in mind when deciding which investigations to order. A blood count, chest x-ray and urine analysis may be requested routinely because they often reveal unsuspected abnormalities. Other tests may have been requested to confirm a provisional diagnosis or to support another, unlisted diagnosis. Tests may be done to assess the severity of a problem, to detect the presence of important complications or to evaluate progress and the effects of therapy. But unfortunately conventional records rarely reveal why investigations were requested, or why individual drugs were prescribed; it is therefore difficult to judge if either the diagnostic work-up or the treatment was appropriate to clinical needs. Comments made to the patient about his illness are rarely recorded even if he is suffering from cancer or from another serious disease.

In the problem orientated system there is a systematic approach to the management of a patient's problems. This helps to avoid serious omissions and to preserve the logic behind the doctor's actions.

Initially we should decide what broad goals are appropriate for the particular patient. This step is especially valuable when caring for the elderly or for those with a terminal illness. For example diagnosis may be eschewed if investigations would cause discomfort or distress or if treatment offers little hope of long or medium term benefit. Broad goals help us to determine priorities when there is conflict over the management of different problems. Often they are obvious and it may seem superfluous to record them. But we should always think about them as they help to keep things in perspective.

A N O   Male   Age 51

5.10.73

PLANS

1   CHRONIC LIVER DISEASE

   Dx - ? chronic active with cirrhosis - no biopsy because of thrombocytopenia
                                          Ba swallow
                                          liver scan

       ? hepatitis B - chronic   HBAg

       ? hepatocellular Ca α feto-protein

   Mx LFTs - monthly

       Urea and electrolytes

       α feto-protein - six-monthly

   RX nil at present
       NB   azathoprine hazardous - thrombocytopenia
            steroids - ? with old TB, ulcer

   Ex Told chronic liver disease - won't get better, but stable at present
       Treatment not indicated yet - but regular review essential

2   THROMBOCYTOPENIA
   Dx   ? 1^0 marrow problem   - bone marrow
                                           haematology consult

   Mx Hb, WBC, indices   )
       platelets   )   monthly
       prothrombin time etc)

   Rx Wait and see
       Must avoid aspirin, phenylbutazone, indomethacin, etc.

   Ex Told about potential hazard of some drugs.   Avoid all drugs unless
       vital. Tell other doctors.   Look out for increased bleeding -
       report if worried.

3   CIGARETTE SMOKING

   Dx   chronic obstructive airways disease - pulmonary function tests
   Ex   must give up or cut down [++]

4   OBESITY
   Rx   1800 cal diet
   Mx   weigh weekly
   Ex   Too heavy. Aim for gradual reduction to 75 Kg over three months

Fig. 2.5 An example of problem orientated plans written initially for the patient whose problem list is presented in **Fig. 2.1a.** Progress notes written several years later are presented in **Fig. 2.7.**

Next we can make a structured plan for individual problems (Fig. 2.5). Each plan should be headed by the number and title of the problem with which it deals. The remainder of the plan has four sub-sections:

1. Collection of further diagnostic information (Dx)
2. Collection of information for monitoring (Mx)

3. Therapy (Rx)
4. Patient education (Ex)

Further diagnostic information (Dx)
After reviewing the data base we may only be able to formulate problems at a low diagnostic level, e.g. 'chest pain', 'weakness of the left leg' or 'splenomegaly'. To make a more precise diagnosis further information must be collected. This may come from relatives and friends, from previous notes or, as a 'secondary history', from the patient; information may also be obtained by further physical examination or from special investigations. The doctor may decide what to collect on the basis of his own prior knowledge, he may ask a more expert colleague or he can refer to a book or a journal.

The information to be collected should be linked in the plans to the corresponding diagnostic hypotheses (*See* Fig. 2.6). Hypotheses (rather than guesses!) are encouraged in plans but they should be likely solutions to the problem under consideration; possibilities which will not be seriously investigated should not be listed. Linking the hypotheses with the evidence collected to support or refute them helps to preserve the logic of the diagnostic process and allows it to be reviewed and evaluated.

```
F C    Male    Age 47

6.7.76

PLANS

STEATORRHOEA

Dx    ? gluten enteropathy    -   jejunal biopsy
                                  serum and red cell folate
                                  Fe and TIBC
      ? bacterial-overgrowth      breath-test
                                  serum B₁₂
                                  barium meal and follow through
      ? pancreatic            -   scan and Lundh test (if biopsy and
                                  breath test normal)

Mx    daily stool weights
      repeat 3 day faecal fat
      Ca, PO₄, Alk Phos

Rx    Nil at present

Ex    Essential to find cause of steatorrhoea.    Likely that therapy
      will then be effective.
```

Fig. 2.6 An example of plans which emphasise the linking of diagnostic hypotheses with the collection of information designed to confirm or refute them. They are not presented as an example of ideal care but to show how the appropriateness of actions can be evaluated.

Information for monitoring (Mx)

Not all new information is collected for diagnostic purposes. Information is also needed to monitor the patient – to help us to decide if a condition is getting better or worse, whether spontaneously or as a result of treatment. Diagnostic tests may only be done once but information for monitoring is usually collected on a number of occasions. Indeed if the patient is suffering from a chronic disease, such as diabetes mellitus, hypertension or chronic renal failure, data will be collected frequently over many years.

It is important that monitoring should be both adequate and appropriate. The incorporation of 'monitoring information' as a separate section of the plans helps to ensure that the process of monitoring receives due consideration. We should record what tests are to be done and the frequency with which they will be requested. Others can then decide whether the plans were appropriate.

Therapy (Rx)

This sub-section should record the treatment which is to be given for the problem under consideration. Surgery, physiotherapy, occupational therapy, etc. should be included here as well as particulars of any drugs prescribed. It is an advantage to record drugs under a problem title as this makes it clear why they were given. The dose, route and frequency of administration should be stated.

When treatment is changed the reason should be clear. When potentially dangerous drugs are administered, e.g. amine-oxidase inhibitors, long term corticosteroids or anticoagulants, there should be a note on the possible hazards and an entry about the drug should be made in the problem list (*See* Figs 2.5, 2.1a and 2.1b).

Patient education (Ex)

This is an extremely important section. Patients frequently complain that they are not told enough about their illnesses and that doctors have too little time to listen to their worries and fears. Such failure of communication is not defensible but it is rarely due to callous indifference on the part of doctors. It happens because it does not always occur to us to spend a few minutes putting our patients' minds at rest. The inclusion of patient education in the basic framework of plans helps to protect against such an oversight.

This section should include a brief description of the information given to the patient about his illness, its management, and its implications for his way of life; it should note the patient's questions or fears, and comments by doctors to relatives should be entered. Those who use the notes need such information because it is sometimes embarrassing and occasionally dangerous not to know what the patient has been told. It is also useful to discuss with patients, and to record, the goals for individual problems. These might include the degree of functional improvement to be sought, in terms of joint mobility or exercise tolerance, or the level to which the blood pressure or body weight should be reduced. Most patients appreciate clarification of the expected response to treatment; their co-operation, and compliance with therapy, may improve as a result.

When a new set of notes is created the initial plans will follow the data base and will in turn be followed by progress notes. When many problems are formulated some may be accorded a low priority and the writing of plans for them may be delayed. Their initial plans can be entered subsequently within the progress notes; it will be easy to find them if the date of entry of the plan is recorded on the problem list.

When a new problem arises relevant clinical details should be recorded in the progress notes together with the plan for this problem. The date of this entry should be listed in the problem list.

Some users of POMR advocate that the initial plan for a problem should recapitulate the data used to formulate the title of the problem e.g. by listing the symptoms, signs and test results which led to the diagnosis of 'congestive heart failure' or 'cirrhosis of the liver'. As this information is already present in the data base it means writing it out a second time. Not surprisingly busy doctors find this a tedious exercise. Indeed it may lead to an unwillingness to formulate problems because of the extra effort involved in writing plans for them.

Progress notes
Follow-up notes are particularly poor in conventional records. Frequently they consist of jottings such as 'better today' or 'no improvement', without reference to the condition commented upon. In simple cases such lack of information may be of little consequence but in complicated cases the importance of good follow-up notes can hardly be exaggerated. Colleagues who are called in to see a patient when the houseman and registrar are off duty may waste a good deal of time trying to acquaint themselves with poor notes, inadequate fluid balance charts, and a jumble of laboratory reports; more often they give up the unequal struggle and either acquire information in other ways or manage the patient on an ad hoc basis giving an opinion without adequate information.

The poor quality of conventional progress notes is due mainly to the lack of an agreed sub-structure as doctors then have no framework to guide them when jotting down their observations and impressions.

The problem orientated structure allows a striking improvement on the chaos of the old system.

A problem orientated progress note is headed by the statement of the problem to which it refers and has four main sub-sections – subjective information (S), objective information (O), assessment (A) and plans (P). The subjective section records *change in the patient's*

A N O   Male Age 54

PROGRESS NOTES

10.4.76   <u>URINARY INFECTION</u>

S̲ Several recent bouts of frequency, burning and fever.
   Clears with Ampicillin. Came off 5 days ago.

O̲ R testicle smaller than L - 2^0 to problem 9.
   Prostate normal size.

P̲ Dx - ? Bladder neck obstruction - IVP
   Mx - CVSU - microsc and culture

1   <u>CHRONIC LIVER DISEASE</u>

S̲ No jaundice, dark urine; ankle swelling worse, no
   swelling, memory good. No vomiting or black stools,
   no itching.

O̲ Liver 3 cm. No bruit. Spleen 4 cm.
   Spiders ++. Oedema → Knees
   No flat or foetor

A̲ Reasonably stable

P̲ Mx - repeat LFTs
   α-FP and HBsAg
   Urea and electrolytes

2   <u>THROMBOCYTOPENIA</u>

S̲ No spontaneous bruising or major bleeds. Occasional
   bleeding nose and gums.

O̲ Petechiae around belt line and 'stasis' petechiae over
   lower legs.

P̲ Mx - Repeat platelets

17.4.76   1   <u>CHRONIC LIVER DISEASE</u>

O̲ Bilirubin 2, AsT 54, Alk Phos 20, Protein 7.0 (Alb 3.1)
   α-FP -ve, HBsAg -ve, Urea 17, K 4.2

A̲ ISQ

P̲ Do nothing

2   <u>THROMBOCYTOPENIA</u>

O̲ Platelets 45 000, WBC 4.5×10^3 (N 33, L 59, E 6, M 2)

5   <u>URINARY INFECTION (+ URETHRAL STRICTURE)</u>

O̲ CVSU   NAD
   IVP - Kidneys normal. Bladder - mild smooth bilobed
   basal prostrate indentation. Micturition urethrography
   irregular narrowing of the urethera.

A̲ Urethral structure → Problem List 44 10

P̲ Dx and Rx - Urological opinion

Fig. 2.7 Examples of Problem Orientated progress notes. They demonstrate how information requested in the planning process is recorded in subsequent progress notes. For further details see text.

symptoms or the absence of an expected change. The objective section describes changes in the patient's signs, and the results of investigations performed to elucidate the problem or help in its management. The third section is a *reassessment* of the problem in the light of the evidence recorded in the two previous sections. *Plans* are made accordingly. These should be sub-structured like initial plans and record decisions about the collection of new information for diagnosis or monitoring, treatment, and patient education. This structured approach helps a doctor to think about several aspects of each problem and provides evidence of whether he has done so. Examples of problem orientated progress notes are shown in Figures 2.7, 2.8 and 2.9.

Progress notes should be brief. Notes need not be made every time the doctor sees the patient; after all they are not written to record whether the doctor has visited, but to record change in the patient's clinical status. When there has been no change, no comment need be made unless the absence of change is itself noteworthy, e.g. a lack of response to treatment. *When writing progress notes, it is not necessary to make an entry for each active problem, nor to write under all four sub-headings.* It

```
P R  Female  Age 68

PROGRESS NOTES

12.3.75      ATRIAL FIB, HYPERTENSION, HEART FAILURE

             S  Dyspnoea improved, no cough or wheezing.  Ankle
                swelling less.

             O  Pulse 100, still irreg.   BP 180/110 (difficult)
                JVP ↑ -3 cm.  Ankle oedema +, slight sacral oedema
                Heart 15 cm, LV +, sounds ISQ

             A  Improving

             P  Rx - Continue bendrofluazide
                                digoxin
                                ∝ methyldopa

14.3.75      ATRIAL FIBRILLATION

             S  Left leg - slight pain noticed 2 hours ago - slightly cold

             O  Skin of left leg slightly pale, cooler than R, no post
                tibal or dorsalis
                Pulse femoral OK, ? popliteal

             A  Embolus to L popliteal

             P  Mx - Observe skin L leg for viability
                         thrombotest

                Rx - Heparin
                     Warfarin
```

Fig. 2.8 An example of progress notes in which several problems listed on the problem list have been incorporated into one heading in order to avoid entering the same data under different problem titles.

N R   Female   Age 42

Problem list includes:

1 Sclerosing cholangitis

2 Ulcerative colitis

8 Xanthomatous neuropathy

14 Visual deterioration

16 Collapse 5th lumbar vertebrae

17 High platelet count

Selected progress Notes

3.1.77 COLLAPSE 5TH LUMBAR V

Mx Urea and electrolytes   )
     serum Ca, PO_4, Alk Phos   ) 2 x / week
     24 hour urine calcium x 3
     Bone biopsy   )
     Skeletal survey   ) for 1:25 Dihydrocholecalciferol (DHC) trial
     Bone densities   )

Rx Bed rest
     Pentazocine 30-60 mg 6 hrly prn
     Diazepam 5 mg qds

6.1.77 COLLAPSE 5TH LUMBAR V

Dx 1.1 cm tetracyline labelled bone from L Iliac crest
     → Histology. Marrow → Haematology (re # 17)

12.1.77 COLLAPSE 5TH LUMBAR V

O Serum Ca 11.7 mg/100 ml
    Urine Ca 75 mg/24 hrs

A In view of high serum Ca not for 1:25 DHC yet

P Rx Orthopaedic opinion - 'lumbar support with mobilisation
        to limit of pain tolerance starting in hydrotherapy
        pool'.

19.1.77 COLLAPSE 5TH LUMBAR V

O Fasting Ca still 11.7 mg/100 ml, PO_4 4.6 on 17.1.77

A ? Related to immobility and previous D_3 therapy
    ∴ Hold off 1.25 DHC. Now more mobile

28.1.77 COLLAPSE 5TH LUMBAR V

S Pain now much better

O Ca 2.6 mmol/l, P 1.26*
    Bone biopsy - severe osteoporosis. No increased osteoid
    Skeletal survey compatible with this, periosteal reaction not
    diagnostically helpful

A No osteomalacia ∴ no indication for 1:25 DHC
    ? Possible that oestrogen deficiency important here

P Dx - 24 hour urinary oestrogen
       Vaginal smear for cells

Fig. 2.9 An example of progress notes in which management was changed in the light of new data. * A change to S I Units took place in the preceding few days.

is a golden rule of POMR that plans and progress notes should be written with economy of words: when there is nothing worth recording nothing should be written!

Some critics of POMR claim that the writing of progress notes under individual problem headings leads to redundancy in the recording of information. This would be true only if closely related problems were documented separately and if items of information relevant to more than one problem were repeated under each heading. When there is overlap between problems it is simpler and more sensible to write combined progress notes with the title of each problem incorporated into the same heading (*See* Fig. 2.8). Reduplication of effort is thus avoided while it is still easy to track individual problems through the progress notes.

If a request for more data is recorded in a plan or progress note then the resulting data should be entered, under the same problem heading, in a subsequent progress note. A reassessment of the problem may be made in the light of the new data and the effect on management evidenced by a change of plans (Fig. 2.9). This structured approach makes it easy to follow the course of each problem and to appreciate the reasons for which decisions are made. This is particularly helpful to a doctor who becomes involved late in an illness or whose involvement is only temporary.

New problems commonly arise during the course of medical care but not all are of major significance. The doctor may not wish to record a headache or abdominal pain on the permanent problem list if he feels

CARDIO-VASCULAR

IN THE PAST YEAR HAVE YOU		YES	NO
1	Had pain or discomfort in your chest lasting more than a minute?	☐	☐
2	Been troubled by skipped or irregular heartbeats or palpitations?	☐	☐
3	Had swollen ankles or feet?	☐	☐
4	Been awakened from sleep with breathlessness or a cough?	☐	☐
5	Had painful leg cramps while walking which forced you to slow down or stop?	☐	☐
6	Had whitening, numbness and/or pain on your fingertips when cold?	☐	☐

HAVE YOU EVER HAD			
7	A heart murmur?	☐	☐
8	A tight or leaky heart valve?	☐	☐
9	Varicose veins?	☐	☐
10	High blood pressure?	☐	☐

Fig. 2.10a Example of questions put to patients in a self administered questionnaire.

CARDIOVASCULAR

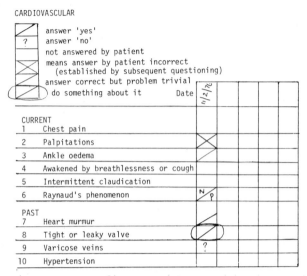

Fig. 2.10b An example of the storage of information obtained from replies to the section of the self administered questionnaire in Fig. 2.10a.

it may be transient or trivial. Such an event can be recorded in the progress notes under the heading of 'temporary problem'.

If a patient is readmitted to hospital with an exacerbation of a condition already present in the problem list details should be recorded in the progress notes. Similarly details about a major new problem can be recorded in progress notes (although some would advocate their inclusion in a separate section of 'histories of presenting complaints'). The problem title would need to be added to the permanent list with a date to tell us where we can find the first entry about it. But with either a new problem or with a serious exacerbation of an old one we might wish to conduct a systems review or check other elements of the defined data base; these can be conveniently recorded in a separate 'data base' section of the notes as illustrated in Figures 2.10b, 3.14.

Flow charts

For certain purposes progress notes are far from ideal. Indeed in emergencies such as diabetic coma, cardiac arrest or gastrointestinal bleeding, narrative progress notes alone are inappropriate and may be counter-productive. They take too long to write and read, and occupy too much space. In such situations rapidly accumulating information may overwhelm us. To prevent this we can use flow charts to record data such as vital signs, laboratory investigations, and details of therapy. Flow charts are simple to use and supply important information at a glance. They are invaluable when the temporal relationship between data is important for their interpretation. Furthermore the time required to initiate a flow sheet is small compared with the time which is otherwise wasted sorting and reassembling disorganised and misplaced data.

When we construct a flow chart we must decide what observations to make and how frequently to make them. Unfortunately there is little information of scientific value to guide us in making these decisions. The general area of monitoring has been sadly neglected. Although laboratory investigations are very costly there are no sensible guidelines on the frequency with which we should carry out tests even in common clinical conditions. But such decisions have to be made and careful deliberations about them may not only benefit the patient but may be of great educational value, particularly to the doctor in training.

A flow chart summarising laboratory data is useful even when the individual results have been recorded in progress notes. Their incorporation in progress notes is beneficial because it allows evaluation of the accompanying 'assessment' and 'plans'. But with a flow chart we can see trends which might be missed on inspection of the individual data. For example a single haemoglobin level of 13 g dl^{-1} would be accepted as normal for a woman; but in juxtaposition to earlier values of 16 g dl^{-1} it might suggest a bleed or an episode of haemolysis. Similarly if the blood urea rose gradually from 3.3 to 6.6 mmol l^{-1} we might search for a cause even though an isolated reading of 6.6 mmol l^{-1} would cause no alarm.

There is another major benefit of the cumulative recording of laboratory results. Individual laboratory report forms can be then removed from the working record and kept in a subsidiary folder. In some patients these forms may add an inch or so to the thickness of the notes and their removal reduces notes to a manageable size.

Some patients with chronic diseases accumulate data slowly but inexorably and the great bulk of their records hampers the review of information, even when they are problem orientated. In such situations flow charts should be used to follow symptoms and physical signs as well as laboratory data. This saves time and paper. Some narrative entries may still be necessary but the progress notes will be much shorter and correspondingly easier to use.

Bjorn and Cross (1970), and others, have designed flow sheets for individual conditions such as hypertension, chronic obstructive airways disease, diabetes mellitus, etc. If a patient has several chronic problems they can each be documented on an individual flow chart;

but Neelon and Ellis (1974) prefer a single flow chart to cover all problems. They argue that separate flow charts obscure interrelationships between problems, and reduce our ability to see the overall course and the response of the 'whole' patient! Furthermore some variables (e.g. weight, pulse rate, blood pressure) have relevance for more than one problem; to record them on separate flow charts would involve reduplication of effort.

If flow charts of any kind are to be used they should be initiated as early as possible in the course of the illness. Ideally they should date from the onset of the problem if the necessary data are available. They can be produced by medical students, trained ancillary staff or may have to be prepared in a doctor's 'spare time'. They may take two minutes to produce, or several hours if volumes of old records are available; in each case we must decide if the expenditure of effort will be worthwhile. Undoubtedly one's understanding of a patient's illness may be drastically improved when a flow chart is constructed and the patient may benefit greatly. The return on the investment comes with every consultation.

THE PROBLEM ORIENTATED SYSTEM

Several ideas about clinical practice are shared by users of problem orientated records and embrace the general areas of comprehensive care, the role of paramedical personnel and nurse practitioners, and the audit of quality of care. They are not the prerogative of users of POMR. Individually they have been advocated for decades, usually by enthusiasts wishing to improve the standards of medical care. But none have been widely accepted despite their apparent attractiveness.

Doctors generally have been reluctant to make the changes necessary to implement these ideas; many feel that they would be deleterious as they threaten traditional methods of practice. But those who use POMR properly have little difficulty in accepting such ideas or in implementing them. Indeed the ideas are logical developments of the principles of POMR outlined earlier in this chapter and the problem orientated record facilitates their implementation. And so instead of the reluctant acceptance of individual ideas, promoted unsuccessfully for many years, there is now a growing willingness to introduce several ideas simultaneously. The resulting pattern of clinical practice has been called the problem orientated system. This 'system' is not clearly defined. Its protagonists would disagree about its boundaries and about the components of the system which would be considered essential. But they would agree about the key role played by the POMR.

Comprehensive care

Traditionally patients have received care for isolated episodes of illness (which may however involve several 'diseases'). In most consultations little or no consideration is given to the 'whole patient'; doctors tend to be interested in other aspects of the patient's health only if they have implications for the management of the major complaints. But we know that the manifestations of some common, serious diseases can be prevented or ameliorated by simple means, e.g. by giving up smoking or alcohol, by losing weight, or by the use of drugs for conditions such as hypertension or hyperuricaemia. If we are to deal effectively with such problems we must know whether our patients smoke, or drink excessively; whether they have asymptomatic hypertension or chronic bronchitis; or whether there are occupational or reversible social factors which might impinge unfavourably on their health. Truly comprehensive care would take such factors into account and ensure not only that important conditions and risk factors are correctly identified but also that they receive appropriate handling.

It is clearly the responsibility of general practitioners to ensure that their patients receive comprehensive care. At present most general practitioners do not exercise this responsibility, excusing themselves on the grounds of pressure of work. Specialists are involved in care on a limited basis; when they are it is important that their activities should be properly co-ordinated into the care of the whole patient.

The problem orientated record facilitates comprehensive care in a number of ways. A correctly constructed problem list includes *all* important problems; it allows us, better than any other means currently available, to 'see' the whole patient and to see each problem in perspective. At every consultation the problem list brings all problems to our attention and we can decide whether one or more of them requires action.

The 'defined' data base also facilitates comprehensive health care. When doctors try to define what information they will collect routinely they recognise the need for a comprehensive collection of data. They also appreciate that the collection of a defined data base can be spread over several consultations; this has obvious implications for a busy practice. But more importantly they realise that by predefining the information which is to be collected routinely they free themselves from the necessity of collecting it personally as it can be collected by questionnaire, or by personnel without a medical qualification or by computer.

A questionnaire is useful for collecting routine elements of the history. Patients can complete it themselves and can take time to do so. They can discuss items with their family and look up old records if necessary. The doctor does not have to spend time asking the many questions which will be answered in the negative; he can use the time saved to elaborate on positive responses, to concentrate on major complaints and to discuss their management and implications with the patient. Sample questions for a self administered questionnaire, and the way in which the answers can be entered into the record are presented in Figures 2.10a and 2.10b.

Paramedical personnel and nurse practitioners

Information from routine physical examination can also be collected without using the doctor's time. For many years nurses, and lay helpers, have recorded patients' weights and heights, and their temperature, pulse rate and blood pressure. They can also be trained to examine the heart, chest, nervous system and pelvic organs. If they are well trained, and perform such examinations frequently, their performance may be better than ours (Alexander, Bloodworth and Orr, 1973).

Such paramedical personnel may be of particular help for the handling of common acute clinical problems, collecting information according to predetermined algorithms or protocols. They collect and record more necessary information than we would normally do ourselves, and reduce the time which doctors need to deal adequately with the patient (Charles *et al*, 1974). They are sometimes allowed to treat minor illness if clear, objective criteria can be defined to guide their actions.

Nurse practitioners are also being used increasingly to supervise the continuing care of common chronic diseases. When the management is relatively straightforward a protocol can be prepared outlining the goals for the problem, the information to be collected at each visit and the indications for change in therapy or for referral back to the doctor. This approach is safe and acceptable to patients and to doctors. Indeed in Burlington, Ontario, nurses have been given a special training, emphasising decision making and clinical judgement rather than procedural skills, and then employed as co-practitioners. They have responsibility to evaluate patient's problems and to choose from three courses of action – specific *treatment*, simple *reassurance*, or *referral* to one of the practice doctors, to another clinician or to an appropriate service agency (Spitzer *et al*, 1974).

The use of paramedical personnel and nurse practitioners has enormous implications for the future of medical care in both rich and poor countries. There is ample precedent for such delegation of clinical responsibility. Midwives work with a great degree of independence, and in specialities such as psychiatry, geriatrics and terminal care, nurses play a major role in patient management. It is now clear that their potential is far greater than has been realised previously and that their role can be extended in a logical fashion. Some doctors will undoubtedly oppose the use of skilled assistants in this way. But it must be emphasised that a doctor's value is not reduced but enhanced if some of his routine functions can be taken over by others: he can then concentrate on the tasks for which his special training is needed, spending more time with the difficult problems of clinical practice and with the control of the quality of the care given to all of his patients, including those seen by nurse practitioners.

The Problem Orientated Medical Record facilitates the use of nurse practitioners and paramedical personnel in patient care. It defines the information which they should collect; it guides what they do subsequently and preserves the logic behind their actions. It also helps doctors to set out their goals and plans clearly so that they can be carried out by others. Many problem orientated practices make successful use of paramedics and nurse practitioners, as described in several chapters in Walker, Hurst and Woody (1973).

Audit

Audit is a key element in the problem orientated system. There is ample evidence that much medical care is of poor quality. Patients may be inadequately or inappropriately investigated and the results may be inaccurate or wrongly interpreted. Treatment is often ineffective and sometimes dangerous. Patients are kept in hospital longer than is necessary. Even the way in which we talk with patients leaves much to be desired.

There are many reasons for poor care. Some are difficult to deal with. But many defects can be corrected by making doctors aware of their existence. This is reflected at a national level, as shown by the consequences of the Confidential Inquiry into Maternal Deaths (Godber, 1976), and also within a single hospital, as evidenced by the change in burst abdomen rates at Guy's Hospital (McColl, 1976). Indeed feedback to doctors about their performance, individually or collectively, must be the most powerful of all influences determining the quality of care.

Audit should be used to provide this feedback; it should not be used in order to punish those who do not match the chosen criteria. Unless audit is seen by doctors as an educational process, helping them to maintain a high level of competence, it will continue to be viewed as a threat to clinical freedom and its widespread introduction in any form will be strongly resisted.

The importance of audit in the problem orientated system cannot be overemphasised. It allows us to check the comprehensiveness of care. We can tell how completely the defined data base has been collected and how thoroughly the problem list has been formulated. We can assess the logic with which plans have been drawn up and how well they have been carried out. Audit allows us to check our performance and correct our deficiencies. We can check the performance of nurse practitioners and paramedical personnel who may be associated with us in the care of our patients; we can give them feedback about their thoroughness and reliability and point out areas in which improvements can be made. Audit is the most important tool for controlling the quality of medical care and as such is the cornerstone of the Problem Orientated System.

A system of audit must be tailored carefully to meet requirements. We can audit the *outcome* of care or the *process* of care. The *outcome* of care depends on many factors: while it is an appropriate measure of the performance of a large specialty group or of an entire hospital it is not a good method for evaluating care given to individual patients or care given by an individual doctor. To do this we must look at the *process* of care to see whether the right things were done. If they were the doctor cannot be blamed for an unfortunate end result.

To audit process, good casenotes are essential. The inadequacy of current medical records for this purpose is widely recognised and many advocate the use of POMR in order to facilitate educational audit. Audit is particularly important during the introduction of POMR (*See* Ch. 5). It is undoubtedly the quickest and most effective way of helping the learner to use POMR correctly. And when audit is used for this purpose the learner instinctively appreciates its value, and that of POMR, for monitoring and so improving the quality of care given to the patient. This, as much as anything, explains the enthusiasm of those who have made genuine attempts to convert their records to a problem orientated format.

CRITICISMS OF THE PROBLEM ORIENTATED RECORD

An American sociologist has claimed that the spread of POMR has followed the pattern of a religious revival. Certainly some of its standard bearers have promoted POMR with missionary zeal and sung its praises with evangelical fervour. Colleagues have reacted in different ways. Some have been convinced that benefits will result from POMR and have converted their own records and/or supported the introduction of POMR into their own hospital or medical school. Many have been less convinced, some have been sceptical, and a few have been openly antagonistic to POMR.

The ballyhoo surrounding the introduction of POMR has contributed to the critical attitude of many doctors. They argue legitimately that enthusiasm for POMR has been based on faith rather than on facts and ask for evidence to support what are sometimes extravagant claims. Such evidence, particularly about quality of care, is hard to come by. There are several reasons for this:

1. To demonstrate that care is better *because* of POMR we must be able to discern differences between the care described in problem orientated notes and that described in notes using a different format. While we can use POMR to assess quality of care, traditional source orientated notes are notoriously inadequate for this purpose. This makes reasonable comparison difficult (if not impossible!)
2. Because doctors have difficulty in converting to POMR many 'problem orientated' records are poor examples of the genre. The potential of POMR for improving care cannot be fully realised with such records; furthermore their defects as casenotes make it difficult to recognise improvements that may have resulted from the partial implementation of the problem orientated approach.
3. Finally it is axiomatic that the correct use of a tool such as the problem orientated record cannot guarantee the quality of the product. Deplorable care could be described perfectly. Clearly, blame for this cannot be placed on the record format. Indeed it would be a major advantage of POMR that the deficiencies in such a record could be spotted easily by another (hopefully abler!) physician and that corrective action might then be taken.

The critics of POMR must receive serious consideration. If they are constructive then their ideas might be incorporated with benefit. Even if they are destructive their comments would be useful if, as a consequence, unsatisfactory elements of POMR were deleted. But spurious criticisms need particular attention; they may sully the climate of opinion about POMR and make it more difficult to convince colleagues of the real benefits which may result from implementation.

Many criticisms of POMR are trivial. Often they appear in editorials or feature articles by writers (not always doctors) who have not used POMR; frequently they misinterpret or misquote their primary sources. With growing interest in POMR more and more of such articles are appearing. Although their criticisms are trivial it is difficult to counter them effectively: readers of these articles may not read further about POMR and will remain unaware of the potential benefits.

Some criticisms are from the pens of highly respected authors and have been published in reputable journals. Most have dealt with limited aspects of the problem orientated record but two of them, by Feinstein (1973) and Goldfinger (1973), have ranged more widely.

Feinstein accepts that POMR have several advantages. He recognises the value of the 'patient profile', and of the inclusion of 'patient education' in the formal structure of plans. He admits that POMR offers a method of arranging complex medical data and concedes that no suitable alternative is currently available. For him its greatest intellectual virtue is that it allows problems to be described in simple terms, so freeing us from the shackles imposed by our conventional taxonomy of disease. Each of these advantages stems from the structure and basic principles of the problem orientated record.

But Feinstein criticises many other aspects of POMR. Almost all of his points can be countered effectively but here I have space to deal only with some of his remarks. He is worried about the definition of a data base or at least about 'the current hypertrophy of the data base . . . without regard to how much of the data is necessary, extraneous or harmful.' Goldfinger, too, is concerned about the data base – with the difficulties of defining a sensible data base; with the idea that the 'data base' should be an elegant, separate entity of the record; and with the reverence with which the data base is regarded, which 'inhibits scepticism and challenge.' The worries of both authors stem from a narrow interpretation of Weed's earlier writings and from their failure to distinguish between problem specific data and the 'defined data base' of routinely collected information. If the 'defined data base' is viewed as a flexible structure (because the choice of items can be left to individual doctors or groups of doctors, and because its content is subject to regular review) then these criticisms are relatively unimportant.

Feinstein is concerned with the effect of POMR on diagnostic reasoning – 'each abnormal finding can be classified directly as a separate problem, and no routine demand is made for diagnostic summations, influences, and explanations.' He could undoubtedly find examples in support of this statement but they would exemplify misuse of POMR and the quotation reveals a poor understanding of the principles of POMR. Diagnostic hypotheses are called for in plans, and appropriate 'tests' should be recorded alongside them (Figs 2.5 and 2.6); a logical approach to the diagnostic process is thus both promoted and preserved in the record. I agree with Feinstein that 'the discipline of providing diagnostic explanations for observed phenomena has been a crux of the skills composing clinical judgement'; but I would argue that it is better served by POMR than by conventional approaches.

Advocates of POMR believe that they help to coordinate activities when more than one doctor looks after a single patient. But Feinstein writes 'the fragmentation of a patient into different specialty zones is often a lamentable flaw of current medical practice, but the problem structured record does not alter this fragmentation. In this record the problem or problems pertinent to each specialty zone are clearly demarcated. Each specialist can approach the chart, find his section of it and augment its data, and depart – without having to be exposed to or to become aware of any problems beyond the boundaries of that specialty.' This is a preposterous proposal which further illustrates Feinstein's poor understanding of POMR (or reflects repeated exposure to its misuse). The problem list allows the visiting specialist to see his own problem in perspective, a facility rarely granted to him with any form of conventional records. Furthermore POMR progress notes should be entered chronologically and a specialist should write after the last entry in the notes – not in a place set aside for his own entries. By doing so he will almost certainly be made aware of the problems which have recently received attention.

Feinstein claims that some of the major 'advantages' of POMR are illusory. He contends that better medical records cannot improve continuity of care; they cannot integrate the activities of health care personnel, cannot serve as an index of quality of care and cannot promote a continuing audit of medical care. He argues that these benefits come 'from either the vigorous supervision needed to make the system work or the previous attitudes of the people who elect to use the system'. But these arguments of Feinstein's are not a matter of dispute. Paradoxically he combines an attack on the problem orientated record with approval of the problem orientated system. Advocates of the system recognise the importance of doctors' attitudes towards the processes of health care; like Feinstein they stress that vigorous supervision is needed to ensure continuity of care, to integrate the activities of health care personnel and to introduce continuing audit of care. Unlike Feinstein they see the problem orientated record as a tool which, when it is used well, allows them to do these things. It is almost impossible to do them without good records.

To assess the work of an individual doctor we need to check what he does for individual patients. Feinstein writes 'The audit involves an evaluation of what has been done *regardless of which way the events are recorded.*' and '. . . audits performed by the supervisor cannot be ascribed to any unique merits of problem-structured data.' But good records are important. Most doctors believe that conventional records are inadequate for the purpose of audit and there is widespread feeling, endorsed by some official bodies (Alment, 1976, Barro, 1973), that *recording* has to be improved if we are to be able to conduct audit effectively.

Supporters of POMR claim that they are superior to conventional records for audit of the quality of care. In a frequently quoted paper Fletcher (1974) questions this claim. House staff were invited to audit problem orientated and source orientated records which contained the same information. There was no difference in the time taken to read each record and answer ten factual questions on its content, nor in the accuracy of the responses to these questions, nor in the proportion of independently determined major errors in medical care recognised in each case history after one reading.

Fletcher's conclusions were vague but he did suggest that medical records were of limited use for assessing the quality of care unless explicit criteria are used. However Feinstein and Goldfinger both gave examples of poor care which are obvious to the reader without explicit criteria having been defined. Surely the main purpose of audit should be to check the analytical sense with which clinical data are handled and not simply conformity to predetermined criteria.

Several features of Fletcher's study were unsatisfactory. First the records used were *artificial* records thus invalidating the test of the hypothesis that 'physicians can audit PORs more rapidly, and with greater accuracy and comprehension, than traditional source orientated records.' Secondly both types of records were prepared from POMR used at the Baltimore City Hospital (and we are not told whether it would have been as easy to prepare them from the source orientated records used at the Johns Hopkins). Thirdly while the problem orientated versions are acceptable, though far from excellent examples of POMR, I would challenge Fletcher's assertion that the examples of source orientated records reflected current practice in Baltimore hospitals. Not only do they contain a 'problem list' but the order of plans corresponded to that of the 'problem list'.

Fletcher's study would have been more helpful if he had tested whether the auditors could tell, from the record, why actions were taken. My own experience using traditional records for this purpose is discouraging – to say the least!

Audit is a matter of crucial importance. If good POMR allows satisfactory audit of the quality of care it would be tragic if articles such as that of Fletcher were to slow down the introduction of POMR and so delay effective audit.

In their criticisms of audit using POMR Feinstein, Goldfinger and others combine to attack a legitimate target. To quote Goldfinger – 'at present, most attempts at audit of records using POMR are designed to measure primarily their style rather than the quality of care delivered.' Carson (1973) claims that 'it is the ability to comply with the system that is "audited" and not the quality of medical care', a point echoed by Field (1974). These critics complain that the style and format of the record are overemphasised and the quality of the content neglected. They also complain that the time necessary for the record keeping impinges on time available for thinking, planning and communicating, while the bibliotechnics of record keeping focus clinical activity on to the record rather than on the patient.

These criticisms are often justified but the fault does not lie with the problem orientated approach. The system is commonly misused because of lack of understanding of the basic principles of problem orientation. There may be redundant information: items within the data base are repeated in the initial plans and progress notes, and extensive narrative notes are written when a flow chart would be better; this wastes time and does impinge on the time available for planning. The notes may not be in chronological order; they may be mixed up with conventional notes; the problem list may be incomplete and initial plans and progress notes unclear, with no reasons given for the collection of information or for treatment. This makes it difficult to follow the notes.

When we try to correct these deficiencies in the use of POMR learners do complain that undue emphasis is placed on the format of the record. But some concentration on style is necessary because the record is a tool; it must be used properly if we are to get the most out of it. When we write a problem orientated medical record correctly the time involved is largely spent on planning and thinking about the patient's problems. It is not wasted on 'record keeping'; planning and thinking are the most important aspects of our work!

When we consider the criticisms of POMR we must ask ourselves whether a suitable alternative exists. Feinstein claimed that the conventional records used during his days as a house officer were good records. 'I have subsequently analysed the data of those records during various formal research projects, and I can vouch for the value of the information. The data were generally well maintained and organised, and a perusal of the medical notes would usually convey a prompt and reasonably clear idea of the patient's major problems at any particular time in his clinical course. Since the records were prepared by human beings they were often imperfect, but the imperfections were usually caused by individual departure from the basic methods and goals. The system itself appeared to work reasonably well.'

I visited Feinstein in November 1974. I wrote in advance to ask him if he would produce some of the records to which he had referred. No examples were produced on arrival or during my three day visit to New Haven. Nor could Feinstein suggest any hospital in the United States where records of the type he mentioned were in use. In view of the current interest in medical records it seems surprising that none of his old colleagues at Yale are capable of producing records up to the old standards.

Should doctors be advised to switch now to POMR, bearing in mind the criticisms mentioned above, and given the problems of implementation which are dealt with more fully in Chapters 3 and 4? I think so. The problem orientated record, when it is properly used, does help us to care for our patients. We are less likely to miss important items of information, to ignore significant problems or to overlook potential interactions; we are less likely to neglect patient education. It is easier to act logically because the record demands that we should give reasons for our actions. All these factors focus our attention on the care of our patients. It cannot make what we do right but it does allow us, and others, to check what we have done. The real importance of the record therefore lies in its content. The good record allows us to assess and improve the quality of our care and it is this, not the style of the record, which justifies change to the problem orientated approach.

ACKNOWLEDGEMENTS

I am grateful to Larry Weed and Geoff Lloyd for their comments on early drafts of this chapter and to them and to Mervyn Maze for many enjoyable hours of discussion on the 'principles of POMR'. John Rhodes and Richard Hunt read the final draft of the chapter and made several helpful suggestions. I must also express my deep gratitude to Sir Francis Avery Jones, to Mr. Geoffrey Phalp, and to the King Edward's Hospital Fund for their support and encouragement of my efforts to promote the Problem Orientated Medical Record.

REFERENCES

Alexander, E. L., Bloodworth, L. P. & Orr, B. T. (1973) in *Applying the Problem Oriented System*, ed. Walker, H. K., Hurst, J. W. & Woody, M. F. Ch. 22, pp. 215–223, New York: Medcom Press.

Alment, E. A. J. (1976) *Competence to Practise*. Report of Committee of Enquiry into Competence to Practise. (Obtainable from 27 Sussex Place, Regents Park, London NW1 4RG).

Barro, A. R. (1973) Survey and Evaluation of Approaches to Physician Performance and Measurement. *Journal of Medical Education.* **48**, 1053–1093.

Bjorn, J. C. & Cross, H. D. (1970) *Problem-oriented Practice*. Chicago: Modern Hospital Press.

Carson, P. (1973) Problem Oriented Medical Record. *British Medical Journal*, **2**, 713.

Charles, G., Stirnson, D. H., Maurier, M. D. & Good, J. C. (1974) Physician's Assistants and Clinical Algorithms in Health Care Delivery - A Case Study. *Annals of Internal Medicine*, **81**, 733–739.

Curtis, P. (1976) New Ideas in Medical Records: Problems of Implementation. *Update*, **12**, 1311–1316.

Feinstein, A. R. (1973) The Problems of the 'Problem-Oriented Medical Record'. *Annals of Internal Medicine*, **78**, 751-762.

Field, M. H. (1974) Problem oriented vs traditional records. *New England Journal of Medicine*, **291**, 108.

Fletcher, R. H. (1974) Auditing Problem-oriented Records and Traditional Records: A controlled comparison of speed, accuracy and identification of errors in medical care. *New England Journal of Medicine*, **290**, 829-833.

Godber, G. (1976) in *A Question of Quality: Roads to assurance in Medical Care*, ed McLachlan, G., pp. 23-33. London, Oxford University Press.

Goldfinger, S. E. (1973) The problem-oriented record: A critique from a believer. *New England Journal of Medicine*, **288**, 606-608.

Hughes, J., Lloyd, G. & McIntyre, N. (1978) The Quality and Educational Value of Medical Records - A Survey of Student Opinion. *Medical Education*, **12**, 267-272.

McColl, I. (1976) in *A Question of Quality: Roads to assurance in medical care*, ed. McLachlan, G. pp. 49-61, London, Oxford University Press.

Neelon, F. A. & Ellis, G. J. (1974) *A Syllabus of Problem-Oriented Care*. Boston: Little, Brown & Co. Ltd.

Pirsig, R. (1974) *Zen and the Art of Motor Cycle Maintenance*, New York: William Morrow and Co., Inc.

Spitzer, W. O., Sackett, D. L., Sibley, J. C., Roberts, R. S., Gent, M., Kergin, D. J., Hackett, B. C. & Olynich, A. (1974) Burlington Randomized Trial of the Nurse Practitioner. *New England Journal of Medicine*, **290**, 251-256.

Tunbridge, R. E. (1965) *The Standardisation of Hospital Medical Records:* Report of the Sub-committee. London, HMSO.

Walker, H. K., Hurst, J. W. & Woody, M. F. (1973) *Applying the Problem-Oriented System*. New York: Medcom Press.

Walker, J. (1967) *Hospital Medical Records in Scotland. Development and Standardisation*: Report of a Sub-committee. Edinburgh, HMSO.

Walker, J. (1973) *Standardisation of Hospital Medical Records*. Report of the Working Party. Edinburgh, HMSO.

Weed, L. L. (1969) *Medical Records, Medical Education and Patient Care*. Chicago: Year Book Medical Publishers.

Weed, L. L. (1975) *Your Health Care and How to Manage it*. Essex Publishing Company, Essex Junction, Vermont, USA.

3

Implementation of the problem orientated medical record in hospital practice

J. C. PETRIE

Senior Lecturer, Department of Therapeutics and Clinical Pharmacology,
University of Aberdeen; Honorary Consultant Physician, Aberdeen Teaching
Hospitals, in collaboration with
Professor W. Walker, Dr. P. D. Bewsher, Dr. D. B. Galloway, Dr. M. Hall,
Dr. W. G. Hendry, Dr. T. A. Jeffers, Dr. H. R. Millar, Dr. L. E.
Murchison, Dr. J. Petersen, Dr. G. R. Petrie, Dr. M. Taylor and Dr. J.
Webster. Department of Therapeutics and Clinical Pharmacology,
Department of Obstetrics and Gynaecology, University of Aberdeen and
Aberdeen Teaching Hospitals.

Records should facilitate care *Avery Jones*

AIM AND BACKGROUND

The aim of this chapter is to discuss the introduction, use, maintenance and extension of the problem orientated medical record (POMR) in hospital practice. A practical, rather than a theoretical approach has been used.

In 1972 the POMR was introduced into our 42-bed acute general medicine ward and outpatient clinic. The experience gained over the last five years by ward and department members, past and present, and by colleagues in other wards, specialties and hospitals forms the basis for the views expressed. Most of our department members who have moved to new posts have introduced, or attempted to introduce, the POMR approach with varying degrees of success and failure. Numerous discussions have also been held with individuals interested in or opposed to the use of POMR.

INTRODUCTION OF POMR TO HOSPITALS

How to start

We strongly recommend introduction of POMR by a small group of individuals as the first step in establishing it. This helps to establish a group of people within the hospital who are familiar with the principles and, equally important, with the common misuses and misunderstandings of POMR. It has been our experience that the best introduction of POMR to potential users is participation in a properly used POMR during a ward round or outpatient clinic. Subsequent discussions about definitions, procedure, objectives, educational theory, scientific evaluation and cost-effectiveness are then more informed and instructive.

Such a limited 'pilot scheme' introduction, with subsequent gradual extension by *informed* individuals, seems an obvious approach because there are many obstacles likely to delay or prevent not only successful simultaneous 'across the hospital' introduction, but more importantly subsequent maintenance of POMR. Limited introduction with gradual extension helps to reduce those difficulties which are due to misuse and misunderstanding of POMR. Obviously, few clinicians are prepared to give support to a new system of recording clinical information which is recommended, or felt to be imposed, by enthusiasts or by a committee of the Health Service or University faculty. If each individual doctor considering the use of POMR is not convinced that there is some merit in assessing for himself its suggested benefits, POMR may be ruled out without even a trial. Limited introduction of POMR retains for the individual consultant the personal decision to use POMR or to reject it. In addition, a sudden switch in record-keeping patterns is avoided. If widespread introduction is attempted and fails, valuable goodwill and resources may be squandered.

Limited introduction of POMR can be done by one individual but maintenance is not feasible when he is off duty or on leave. Introduction by a 'firm' or 'team' is the best way to start. Experiments with and modifications of stationery can be made without undue consultation and users have a feeling of participation rather than of obligation. Experience is gained of practical difficulties and solutions are sought from more experienced users, or from the literature on POMR, otherwise prejudice forms against the use of POMR because of the appearance of badly written and executed POMR notes which are the result of errors of understanding of its principles or format. Such notes are common and do a disservice to possible acceptance, use, maintenance and extension of POMR.

Our own first impressions of using POMR were that the problem list (Fig. 3.1) was invaluable and that patients appeared to appreciate our ability to recall their problems. However, a considerable investment of time was required to peruse the contents of the entire 'old' record to create a reliable and accurate problem list. Of course such a perusal of the record should be done in caring for patients with any alternative system. Fortunately, the initial investment of time needed to create the record was seen, by both junior and senior medical and nursing staff, to be repaid each time the record was used.

Most junior staff also appreciated the greater or more apparent opportunity to be managers, planners and doctors during the collection of information and formulation of problems and plans (diagnostic, monitoring, therapeutic and patient education) for each active problem. In general they also welcomed the more frequent, constructive advice from more senior staff about the reliability of their findings, and about their analytical sense in creating the list of problems and the plans for each problem. We found that up to six weeks of participation in the writing of POMR notes was needed by most newcomers to the system to appreciate most of the conceptual and practical aspects of the POMR system and to write useful and economical entries in the notes.

In our experience, once the initial decision had been made to assess the implications for our team of the introduction of POMR we soon overcame much of our initial hostility and became increasingly committed to the gradual conversion of all our case records to POMR starting with all current inpatient case records, with subsequent extension to the case records of patients attending the outpatient clinics.

This move to POMR occurred despite our belief that not all old 'traditional' records are bad. Some are excellent and well suited to the needs and practices of individual clinicians. However, such records are seldom capable of extension, or use and maintenance by other individuals or hospitals, because of the 'individualistic' component, and because of the lack of defined procedural guidelines which new users of the record can follow and use.

Use and maintenance

The principles of POMR are straightforward and have been described in earlier chapters. But consideration of the principles without attention to the real and practical problems of implementation is naïve. Some of the important points which must be kept in mind and which arise during discussions about the writing of case records and about the use, misuse and maintenance of a POMR system in clinical practice are discussed below. Failure fully to appreciate these *separate* points leads in our experience to misunderstanding, misuse, and possibly collapse of a functioning POMR.

— Listen to the patient. Maintain the doctor-patient relationship.

— A sound case history and examination remain the basis of diagnosis.

— Any system of note keeping, including POMR, is only as good as the competence of the individuals who contribute to it. Supervision is essential.

— Always consider the whole patient, not just fragments. The patient is more than the the sum of his problem list, however expertly constructed.

— Do not lose sight of the principal presenting complaint. Structure and subdivisions can feed on themselves and lose their centre of reference.

— Slavish adherence to the entire POMR guidelines, for example *always* making an entry under each separate heading of S.O.A.P., is not essential and is a misuse of the system. This is discussed further in this chapter and in Chapter 2.

— There is a point where further and repetitive discussion of procedural details becomes unproductive or counterproductive. This can act as a disadvantage to offset other advantages. The form of the notes must not be over-emphasised to the detriment of the overall care of the patient. This is a misuse of the system. A balance is *not* difficult to achieve if the difficulty is borne in mind.

— Without supervision, or with only occasional casual participation by senior staff in hospitals, the POMR system is unreliable and inefficient because of the lack, or absence, of quality control. Such an uncontrolled system may give a false sense of security and is perhaps worse than a traditional system which one can't trust at all because undue reliance may be placed on a problem list which is, by default, incomplete and inaccurate. If problems are 'hidden' or 'lost' this inevitably results in a failure by the doctor to recognise 'events' and to report his predictable misadventures. In such a poorly supervised system the contents of the case record should therefore be perused thoroughly at each contact with the patient to make sure that iatrogenic disease is not being caused unwittingly because of ignorance on the doctor's part of risk factors, of organ dysfunction, or of major problems which are not recorded on the problem list. We have noted that such disordered records are sometimes ignored.

— Many doctors regard the problem list as the main but modest advantage of POMR. But doctors who use only the problem list *do not understand* the system. *This is not problem-orientation.* A good history, a defined routine data base, definition of problems, formulation of plans and *supervision* and critical assessment of the collection of information and performance of the individual user are essential to obtain the full practical, educational and conceptual benefits.

— The active interest of senior doctors in supervision of the performance of juniors using the system is a small price to pay for the benefits which accrue to both senior and junior staff. Junior staff quickly become discouraged if their carefully thought out notes and plans are ignored. They ask themselves 'why write anything at all under such circumstances?'

— It is essential that continuing education is provided about the *conceptual* and *practical* aspects of POMR. Junior staff and students move to new posts at frequent intervals and the continuity and smooth usage and maintenance of POMR are disrupted if newcomers do not understand the implications of their contribution. Senior staff care for individual patients with problem-orientated notes for years. It is in their interest that high standards of accuracy are maintained when staff move to new posts. Indeed, junior staff may not be the individuals who benefit most in the overall time saving which we believe accrues over the years.

— Registrars, senior house officers and house officers should not waste time rewriting, in their own hand, yet another case history which has already been recorded by their junior. Instead they should discuss and refine both the information collected and the plans. In other words they should audit the reliability, thoroughness, efficiency and analytical sense of their junior. This may also include audit of the performance of senior medical students who, in our wards, are asked to compile the formal case notes during their eight weeks full-time clinical attachments in medicine and obstetrics and gynaecology. Such supervision – or audit – also occurs with the use of traditional systems of case note recording but is usually more explicit and formalised with POMR because of the defined procedural guidelines. We have found that senior staff are able to assess more quickly the level of performance of which juniors are capable because plans are written along defined guidelines when relevant, for each active problem, under a clear heading, e.g. *7. Diabetes mellitus.*

— We have also found that in the early stages of using POMR, newcomers seem to feel that fragmentation of problems is necessary, rather than interpretation and synthesis. For example dyspnoea and ankle swelling may be listed separately even though the user knows that both are manifestations of congestive cardiac failure. This fragmentation is undesirable and is a misuse of the system.

— Junior staff should not be expected to write all the follow up notes while senior staff hold back. Most junior staff also resent having to write out longhand, repeatedly, similar items of routine information (family history, systematic enquiry, physical examination) on each admission or readmission. Nevertheless, this time wasting, often poorly legible work continues in some wards.

— The interface between those clinicians who keep POMR notes and those who do not is difficult. A threat may be posed, especially when the care of a patient overlaps several specialties. In addition, sharing of care may interrupt the evolution of notes in a sequential POMR format. Alternatively, the patient may be admitted to hospital to the care of clinicians who do not use the POMR system, and the problem list ignored. In such cases it should be updated at the subsequent contact with the patient.

— Whatever the records system, increased secretarial resources are desirable though not, beyond a reasonable level of adequacy, essential. POMR does not, in itself, require additional allocation of secretarial resources.

In addition to these general points about the *use* and *maintenance* of a POMR system in hospitals a number of *specific* points of clarification about the introduction and use of the different components of the POMR system may be helpful.

The data base
History of presenting complaints. We impose no restrictions on the classical system of history taking. Our sheets are only partly structured and much blank paper is provided (Fig. 3.3)
Collection of routine information (defined data base). Each individual in the team should be given the opportunity to draw up his personal requirement of the minimum information to be collected routinely from each patient seen as an inpatient or outpatient. The different contributions should be brought together and circulated to all members of the team. After some discussion a form is typed, then photocopied and used as a short-term, defined routine data base.

ABERDEEN HOSPITALS   MASTER PROBLEM LIST

Addressograph space

Names .... Jane SMITH ....   Unit Number .. 123456 ....

(instructions on use — P.T.O.)

PROBLEM NUMBER	ACTIVE PROBLEMS Include Symptoms, Signs and Abnormal Investigations not Explained by Another Entry. Social and Psychiatric Problems Should Also Be Included.	DATE ENTERED	INACTIVE PROBLEMS Include Major Past Illness, Operations or Hypersensitivities. Do Not Include Problems for Which You Will Provide Active Care.	DATE ENTERED
1			Appendicectomy (1931)	1.6.74
2	Smoking (1939)	1.6.74	→	2.2.75
3	Obesity (1960)	1.6.74	→	3.11.76
4	Varicose veins	1.6.74	~~Surgery (1949)~~ Ligation and stripping (1949)	1.6.74 15.6.74
5			Back pain (1959)	1.6.74
6	Diabetes mellitus maturity onset (1965)	1.6.74		
7	Cataract, rt. eye 2° # 6	1.6.74		
8	Social, lives alone	1.6.74		
9	Myocardial infarction (1974)	2.6.74		
10				
11				
12				
13				
14				
15				
16				

S311

Fig. 3.1 Problem list (master or permanent). Note the date of diagnosis, the date of entry of the problem title in the problem list, the amendment of a title (4) and the use of the arrow to change the status of a problem from active → inactive are shown (2 and 3).

PROBLEM ORIENTATED MEDICAL RECORDS

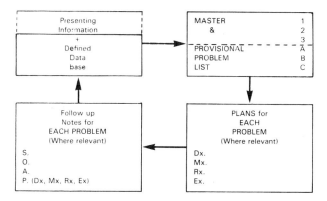

1. A **problem** includes anything which is relevant to the care of the patient.

2. The principal presenting complaint must be clearly stated. The systematic enquiry, physical examination and routine tests constitute the **defined** DATA BASE. This varies from specialty to specialty and ward to ward.

3. **MASTER PROBLEM LIST** entries should be restricted to clear-cut diagnoses or problems, preferably in chronological order, e.g. 6. Diabetes mellitus, chemical (1964) 17.6.'78.
   This list should **always** be regarded as incomplete.
   The numbering of problems should **not** be changed.
   There should be only **one** master problem list always filed at the front of each folder.
   PROVISIONAL PROBLEM LIST entries are provisional diagnoses, evolving problems, guesses, signs or tests of uncertain meaning. If the problem is resolved the master and provisional lists should be revised, with dates, e.g.
17/6 A.	chest pain → 1.	21.6.78.
17/6 B.	Systolic murmur → close.	21.6.78.
17/6 C.	Incomplete data base → close.	24.6.78.

4. **PLANS.** These have **guidelines** which need **not** be slavishly adhered to each time an entry is made. The guideline for an **initial** plan is
A Chest pain	Dx	further data for diagnosis
	Mx	further data for monitoring
	Rx	therapy
	Ex	plans for education of patient

5. **Follow up notes.** These also have structured guidelines
e.g. **4 Diabetes mellitus**	(S)	Subjective data
	(O)	Objective data including investigations
	(A)	Assessment
	(P)	Plans (Dx, Mx, Rx, Ex)
   Entries may be written across a page
   e.g. **6 Obesity** Mx. Weight daily . . . . . . Ex . . . . . .

6. **DISCHARGE SUMMARY.** The principal 'active' problems should be commented on **in order of priority** for the admission. A clear statement of the **plans** for each of these problems should be made.
   Coding for SMR1 is taken from the order of discussion and **not** from the master problem list.

Fig. 3.2 Reverse side of problem list shown in Figure 3.1. The reminder, present in all records, of the procedural details of POMR has been very helpful.

ABERDEEN HOSPITALS		GENERAL MEDICINE — IN PATIENT		
Consultant DR. JONES	Patient's Surname SMITH		Unit Number 123456	
Ward/Dept. 4, A.F.I.	First Names Jane			
Date of Admission 1.6.74	Age 67	Occupation		
	Affix label in box	House Officer J. Brown		

COMPLAINT
  Chest pain

DURATION   ALLERGIES   None
  3 hours

HISTORY OF PRESENT ILLNESS   DRUGS   Morphine
                                                         metformin
                                                         glyceryl trinitrate

> Woke at 3.00 a.m. with severe anterior chest pain
> which persisted for 3 hours until given morphine
> i.m. by G.P.

> Pain radiated down left arm and into jaw. Associated
> with faintness, profuse sweating, nausea and one episode
> of vomiting.

> Has had chest pain on exertion for about 5 years – pain
> of similar character but much less severe and relieved
> by glyceryl trinitrate. Exercise tolerance 100 yards
> on flat, or 1 flight of stairs. Also mild exertional
> dyspnoea for a few years but no orthopnoea or paroxysmal
> nocturnal dyspnoea.

> For many years has had varicose veins and mild ankle
> swelling.

> No palpitations or claudication.

S.26
P.O.M.R. (FILE IN SECTION "B")

Fig. 3.3 History of presenting illness sheet used in medical wards.

PREVIOUS MEDICAL HISTORY
Including:- Rheumatic Fever; T.B.; Diabetes; Jaundice; Operations; Accidents;
          Pregnancies; Transfusions; Mental Illness.

FAMILY HISTORY
Including:- Diabetes, Hypertension, Heart Disease, T.B.

Father
Mother
Sibs
Spouse
Children

SOCIAL HISTORY
Marital Status
Occupation
Husband's Occupation
Dependent Relatives
Home Assistance
Home Conditions
Foreign Residence
Tobacco
Alcohol

PATIENT PROFILE

ROUTINE INVESTIGATIONS

Hb	Urea	ECG
Differential	Na	Chest X-ray
White Cell Count	K	Urinalysis
Film	HCO_3	FOB
ESR		

Fig. 3.4 Reverse side of sheet shown in Figure 3.3. This is the first sheet of the routine, defined data base (medical).

ABERDEEN HOSPITALS

Consultant	Patient's Surname		Unit Number
Ward/Dept.	First Names		
Date	Age	Occupation	

Affix label in box

SYSTEMATIC ENQUIRY		CNS cont	Sensation
			Vision
RS	Cough		Diplopia
	Sputum		Hearing
	Haemoptysis		Mood
	Wheeze		Memory
	Sinusitis	HS	Bleeding/bruising/rashes
	Night sweats		Tongue
	Chest pain	ES	Heat tolerance
CVS	Angina		Xs sweating
	Dyspnoea — rest		Neck swelling
	— exercise		Voice change
	— nocturnal		Irritability
	— orthopnoea		Tremor
	Palpitations		Thirst
	Ankle swelling		Pruritus
	Varicose veins	LS	Joint symptoms
	Claudication		
	Other		PHYSICAL EXAMINATION
GIS	Appetite		
	Weight		General
	Dysphagia		
	Nausea		
	Vomiting		Weight
	Haematemesis		Temp.
	Heartburn		Facies
	Dyspepsia		Pallor
	Fat intolerance		Skin
	Flatulence		Mucous membranes
	Jaundice		Cyanosis central
	Abd. pain		peripheral
	Constipation		Teeth
	Diarrhoea		Tongue
	Piles		Fauces
	Melaena		Jaundice
	Stool		Pigment
	Rectal bleeding		Clubbing
GUS	Dysuria		Koilonychia
	Nocturia		Thyroid
	Haematuria		Breasts
	Frequency		Nodes
	Difficulty		Other
	Stream	RS	Sputum
	Dribbling		Tachypnoea
	Incontinence		Access. muscles
	LMP		Chest shape
	Discharge		Trachea
	P.M. bleeding		Mvt.
CNS	Headaches		Expansion
	Dizziness		Percussion
	Fits		Fremitus
	Fainting		Air entry
	Vertigo		Breath sounds
	Ataxia		Added sounds
	Weakness		Voc. resonance

Fig. 3.5 Defined data base, second sheet (medical).

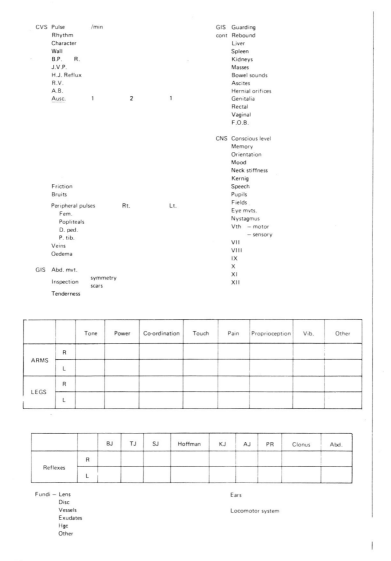

CVS	Pulse	/min				GIS	Guarding
	Rhythm					cont	Rebound
	Character						Liver
	Wall						Spleen
	B.P. R.						Kidneys
	J.V.P.						Masses
	H.J. Reflux						Bowel sounds
	R.V.						Ascites
	A.B.						Hernial orifices
	Ausc.	1	2	1			Genitalia
							Rectal
							Vaginal
							F.O.B.

CNS Conscious level
Memory
Orientation
Mood
Neck stiffness
Kernig
Friction   Speech
Bruits   Pupils
                          Fields
Peripheral pulses Rt.   Lt.   Eye mvts.
  Fem.   Nystagmus
  Popliteals   Vth — motor
  D. ped.   — sensory
  P. tib.   VII
Veins   VIII
Oedema   IX
                         X
GIS Abd. mvt.   XI
                         XII
     Inspection symmetry
                 scars
     Tenderness

		Tone	Power	Co-ordination	Touch	Pain	Proprioception	Vib.	Other
ARMS	R								
	L								
LEGS	R								
	L								

		BJ	TJ	SJ	Hoffman	KJ	AJ	PR	Clonus	Abd.
Reflexes	R									
	L									

Fundi — Lens   Ears
        Disc
        Vessels   Locomotor system
        Exudates
        Hge
        Other

Fig. 3.6 Reverse side of sheet shown in Figure 3.5. Defined data base, third sheet (medical).

ABERDEEN HOSPITALS

Consultant	Patient's Surname	Unit Number
	SMITH	123466
Ward/Dept.	First Names	
	Jane	
	Age	Occupation
		Affix label in box

PROVISIONAL PROBLEM LIST

Date		Problem	Resolved	Date Resolved	Date		Problem	Resolved	Date Resolved
1.6.74	A	Chest pain	→ 9	2.6.74		G			
1.6.74	B	Pallor	→ close	2.6.74		H			
1.6.74	C	Incomplete data base		14.6.74		I			
4.6.74	D	Urea raised	→ close	14.6.74		J			
	E					K			
	F					L			

DATE

1.6.74   **A. Chest pain**

      Dx ? myocardial infarction and cardiac failure – Asp.AT.
      Mx Serial ECGs, cardiorater, i.v. line. Check fluid balance.
      Rx Bed rest, oxygen.
           Bumetanide, see drug cardex.
      Ex Told that probable heart attack, reassured.

2. Smoking

      Ex Advised to stop!

3. Obesity   Plan.

      Rx 1000 calorie diet. Dietician to see later.
      Ex Told aggravating diabetes, and possibly contributing to A. chest pain.

6. Diabetes   Plan.

      Mx Glycosuria chart. Blood sugar 2 hours p.c.
      Rx Continue present metformin – see cardex

8. Social   Plan. & Ex Get social worker to see.

B. Pallor

      Dx ? Associated with A. chest pain. Await data base Hb. result.

2.6.74   **A. Chest pain**

      S. No recurrence of pain. O clear E.C.G. evidence of myocardial infarction. Also Asp.AT 53. p. 70/min., triple rhythm. Basal creps.
    Plan Mx Stop cardiorater; stop i.v. line
      Ex Told that definite heart attack. Given explanatory booklet.

B. Pallor

      O Hb. 13 gm. F.O.B. –ve. Plan. Close.

Fig. 3.7 Provisional problem list and initial plans. The provisional problems are lettered. Note that the use of the date columns help the user to find the relevant entry in the follow up notes. (cross-reference to Fig. 3.1).

ABERDEEN HOSPITALS General Medicine P.O.M.R. Summary Sheet	PATIENT'S NAME AND ADDRESS:			Unit No.
				D. of B.

Occupation			Marital State:

Ward	Hospital		Consultant
Date pl. on W.L.	Transferred from		Referred by
Admitted	Discharged		Disposal

G.P.

PRESENTING MEDICAL HISTORY   WEIGHT

FAMILY & SOCIAL HISTORY

Medicines prior to admission

EXAMINATION

INVESTIGATION RESULTS (Positive or relevant negative)

SIDE ROOM	ESR	FOB
Urine	Sp.Gr...............Sugar................... Alb...................Micro	
Bacteriology & Biochemistry		
Radiology and Electrocardiography		
Haematology & other		

S.28 AM
P.O.M.R. MEDICAL RECORDS COPY

Fig. 3.8 Discharge summary, side 1, medical.

PROBLEM LIST 'CHRONOLOGICAL (Active or Inactive)

ACTIVE		INACTIVE	
		1. Appendicectomy (1931)	
2. Smoking (1939)			
3. Obesity (1960)			
4. Varicose veins		4.1 Ligation and stripping (1949)	
		5. Back pain (1959)	
6. Diabetes mellitus – – maturity onset (1965)			
7. Cataract, rt. eye – – 2° to 6			
8. Social			
9. Myocardial infarction (1974)			

Code	PROBLEM NO. and Title: Assessment, Progress, Plans - Therapy, Patient Education. (Comment in order of priority).

9. Myocardial Infarction – The presenting symptoms were due to an antero-septal infarction, complicated by mild left ventricular failure which responded to bumetanide. Her progress in the ward was uneventful. She is aware that she has had a heart attack. She is on no therapy and no follow-up is proposed.

6. Diabetes Mellitus – She continues on metformin 1.5 gm/day. An appointment has been made at the Diabetic Clinic in 6 weeks' time.

3. Obesity – On discharge 75 kg. She has been given dietary advice.

8. Social – This may prove to be the eventual major problem. She lives alone, up 36 steps. She has been transferred to the convalescent hospital for 3 weeks. The medical social worker is in touch with the relatives.

2. Smoking – This must stop!

Histology of Tumour	1. verified 2. verification pending 3. not requested	Tumour Type	

MEDICINES ADMINISTERED

Oxygen, bumetanide

ADVERSE EFFECTS OF MEDICINES (for reporting to the Committee on Safety of Medicines)

None

Follow-up Plan & Recommended Therapy

Metformin 1.5 gm/day
Diabetic Clinic - 6 weeks.

Copies to: Diabetic Clinic

Signature ABE.R.DEEN Date 15.6.74

Status Registrar

Fig. 3.9 Discharge summary, side 2, medical (cross reference to Figs 3.1; 3.7).

GRAMPIAN HEALTH BOARD

A   66853

Dear Dr. ....
    Your patient was discharged on ....
    It is recommended that the following therapy be continued. A3/ .... days supply has/has not been dispensed.

Problem No.	Medicine and Type of Preparation	Dose	Times of Administration				Method of Administration	Quantity Supplied

Drug/Medicine Sensitivity

Date dispensed......................... Pharmacist's Initials.....................

OTHER TREATMENT AND COMMENTS:

House Officer..

A discharge letter/summary will follow

This copy to be sent to G.P.

S.81

Fig. 3.10 Medication on discharge sheet (N.C.R. copies to notes and to Pharmacy).

Criticism of the information items specified in the data base should be invited and welcomed and the data base sheets amended. After some weeks the sheets showing the agreed minimum requirement of information should be printed because their acceptability to users is increased.

A common misunderstanding is that the defined routine data base must be the same for all units. This is incorrect. Each unit or specialty group should define their own agreed minimum amount of information which they require to be collected from each patient (see Figs. 3.4, 3.5, 3.6, 3.11, 3.12, 3.13, 3.14). In our experience incomplete and poor quality collection of information results if too much routine information is requested.

Space is provided on our data base sheets alongside each symptom for minor comments (Figs. 3.4, 3.5, 3.6). If this space is inadequate for

ABERDEEN HOSPITALS

Consultant	Patient's Surname		Unit Number
Ward/Dept.	First Names		
Date	Age	Occupation	

Affix label in box

SYSTEMATIC ENQUIRY

RS
Cough
Sputum
Haemoptysis
Wheeze
Chest pain
Smoking

CVS
Angina
Dyspnoea — rest
        exercise
        orthopnoea
Palpitations
Ankle swelling
Claudication
Varicose veins

GIS
Appetite
Weight
Dysphagia
Nausea
Vomiting
Heartburn
Haematemesis
Flatulence
Fat intolerance
Jaundice
Abdominal pain
Constipation
Diarrhoea
Piles
Melaena
Stool
PR bleeding

GUS
Loin pain
Dysuria
Nocturia
Frequency
Haematuria
Dribbling
Stream
Difficulty

GUS cont'd
Incontinence
LMP
PM bleeding
Discharge

CNS Headaches
Fits
Depression

ES Bleeding/bruising/rashes
Neck swelling
Sweating
Thirst
Pruritus

Joint symptoms

Alcohol

PHYSICAL EXAMINATION

General

Weight
Temperature
Pallor
Skin
Mucous membranes
Cyanosis
Jaundice
Tongue
Nails
Thyroid

Breasts

Nodes

RS Sputum
Resp rate
Trachea
Movement
Expansion
Percussion
Air entry
Breath sounds
Added sounds

P.O.M.R.
S 309 S   (FILE IN SECTION "B")

Fig. 3.11 Example of data base sheet, surgery.

ABERDEEN HOSPITALS | Gynaecological Systematic Enquiry

Date:

Patient's Surname | Unit Number

MENSTRUATION

Age at Menarche (yrs.)

Date of L.M.P.

First Names

Gestation if pregnant (wks.)

Age | Occupation

Usual Menstrual Cycle (days)

Variation........................

Menorrhagia...

Intermenstrual Bleeding ....

Post Coital Bleeding ....

Post Menopausal Bleeding ....

Dysmenorrhoea: Primary ....

Secondary ....

Other ....

URINARY SYMPTOMS

None ....

Frequency ....

Dysuria ....

Haematuria ....

Stress Incontinence ....

Urgency........................

Urge Incontinence ....

Total Incontinence ....

Delay in starting ....

Other ....

CONTRACEPTION

Method

	From	To
None		
Oral		
I.U.C.D.		
Diaphragm........		
Condom.........		
Coitus Interruptus.........		
Rhythm...........		
Sterilised		
Vasectomy		
(date:		
Other		

Comment ....

PAIN

None ....

Suprapubic.....................

Iliac Fossa ....

Loin ....

Backache ....

Other (specify)......................

MISCELLANEOUS

Vaginal discharge (describe) ....

Pruritis vulvae......................

"Something coming down" ....

Flushings......................

Abdominal distension ....

Hirsuties......................

Infertility: Primary ....

Secondary......................

Other......................

Reproductive Plans

Wants more children........................

Wants contraceptive advice ....

Wants sterilisation ....

Doesn't know ....

SEXUAL UPSET

None........................

Inactive......................

Apareunia ....

Dyspareunia: Deep ....

Superficial.......................

Loss of Libido ....

Other.........................

S.33 (FILE IN SECTION "B")

Fig. 3.12 Example of data base sheet, gynaecology.

BOOKING ARRANGEMENTS			SURNAME	UNIT NUMBER
ANTENATAL CARE	Tick	Note		
Specialist Hospital Clinic			FIRST NAMES	
Consultant			DATE OF BIRTH	
Other Clinic				
Combined Care			ADDRESSOGRAPH PANEL	
General Practitioner			WARD	
Consultation Only			CONSULTANT	

DELIVERY		
Specialist Hospital		
Consultant Only		
Other Hospital		
Domiciliary		
Early Discharge		
Previous Booking		

POST NATAL		
Specialist Hospital		
Other Clinic		
General Practitioner		

ADMISSION AND DISCHARGE DATA

MOTHER ADMITTED				DISCHARGED			TO ATTEND	
Date	From	To	Type	Date	From	To	Clinic	Date
INFANT								

SUMMARY OF PRESENT PREGNANCY

Date	Place	Labour and Delivery							Complications
		Gest. wks.	certain/ uncertain	Onset Sp/Ind	Dur. Hrs.	Oxy. Drip	Delivery	PPS	

Infant	Sex	Weight	LB/SB/1st week death	Name	Unit No.

PERINATAL DEATH	CLINOPATHOLOGICAL CLASSIFICATION
Cause of death as detailed on Death Certificate	
I a	
b	
c	
II	
AMH.51	

Fig. 3.13 Example of data base sheet, obstetrics.

	Day					Day			
	Month					Month			
	Year					Year			

NEUROLOGICAL, MUSCULAR AND SKELETAL (continued)

SOCIAL (continued)

Current

Muscle weakness

Walking aids

Past

Loss of vision

Severe pain - neck/shoulder/arm

Severe pain - back/hip/leg

b) problems in relationship
  -wants help

Problems with children
  -wants help

Family arguments/problems
  -wants help

Death/illness in family/friends

a) Self-employed

b) Employed

c) Housewife

d) Student

e) Pensioner

f) Retired

g) Unemployed

Occupation

SKIN

Current

Rashes

Pruritus

Change in mole(s)

Past

Recurrent boils

BLOOD

Current

Prolonged bleeding

Bruising w/o adequate cause

Occupational hazards/risks

SOCIAL

Previous jobs

Lives

a) alone

b) with parents

c) with spouse/partner

d) with children

e) with other relatives

f) with friends

g) other

Marital status

If working

a) hours worked/week

b) unhappy-working hours

c) dissatisfying job

d) unhappy-working conditions

e) total travelling time/hours

f) finds travel tiring

g) job change actual/ contemplated

h) time in present job months/years

Change in marital status

If Married/cohabiting

a) spouse's occupation

Fig. 3.14 Example of data sheet, medical, showing use of columns. (Royal Free Hospital, London).

comment the problem is elaborated under a problem heading in the follow up notes. Some have suggested a series of columns alongside each symptom in the data base sheets for use during readmissions (for example, Fig. 3.14). We do not favour this because of the restriction on space and because we believe that it is irritating to have to go backwards in the records from the new progress notes to find the original sheet during subsequent admissions. We prefer to use a new systematic enquiry/physical examination sheet (Figs. 3.5, 3.6) for each readmission. However, we do *not* repeat the section in the case history devoted to previous medical history, family and social history (Fig. 3.4). Instead its current accuracy is verified by discussion with the patient.

Often, for various reasons all the defined, routine information *cannot* be collected at the time of the first contact with the patient. In such cases an entry is made on the problem list, i.e. Problem = incomplete data base (Fig. 3.7). This is a most useful practical point. When time or clinical conditions permit the omission is rectified and the problem list is revised.

Check lists or pre-printed sheets are not exclusive to POMR. We have found that legibility is improved, and that the sheets help to identify rapidly what information has been gathered, and equally important, has *not* been gathered.

One common misunderstanding is that questions must be asked in the order of appearance in the defined information section of the data base. Our resident staff often taken the case history, carry out the physical examination and subsequently complete the forms. Not infrequently they are reminded, because of the pre-printed sheets, of omissions.

The use of printed history/examination forms by students has also been criticised as encouraging a 'check list' approach to clinical medicine. We accept this as a risk if used carelessly, but feel that this risk is generally outweighed by the training of students to a methodical and analytical approach to patient care. We stress the importance of careful history taking and meticulous examination and encourage students to talk to the patient. Printed forms need not be taken to the bedside – indeed, students find that later transcription of case histories to printed forms can serve as a valuable feedback on their own thoroughness and developing clinical skills.

The section in our data base which is set aside for a description of the patient profile (Fig. 3.4 and Ch. 2) is essential to good management. However, we have not yet succeeded in defining precisely what information to collect. Usually a description of the life style and social factors is recorded.

A routine number of investigations to be carried out on each patient have also been agreed by our team (Fig. 3.4). Our house staff and students do *not* include such investigations in their initial plans for specific problems.

We have recently started to give pre-printed questionnaires to hypertensive patients to complete outside valuable clinic time. These questionnaires are *not* specific to POMR and are discussed elsewhere in this volume. It is obvious that the information must be confirmed with the patient at interview.

Problem lists

In our experience this aspect of POMR presents few difficulties. Nevertheless, certain practical points deserve emphasis.

The master problem list. The master (or permanent) problem list (Fig. 3.1) should *always* be regarded as incomplete, at least until a discharge summary has been completed. It is essential that the provisional problem list (Fig. 3.7) is also always checked for the presence of additional, active, evolving and as yet ill-defined problems.

Straightforward problem titles or diagnoses (e.g. obesity, smoking) should be entered directly on the master problem list by the person taking the history. Any clearly descriptive problem title is appropriate. We prefer that some chronological order is used because important new problems can be added as the list grows. However, a strict chronological sequence is not essential.

Less well defined entries, guesses or unsubstantiated diagnoses, or signs are entered in a simple descriptive manner in the provisional problem list. With both categories of problem we try to record the date that the problem was first diagnosed because this is useful information if it is immediately available. We insist that the first date of entry of the problem in the record is recorded. This should permit easy reference to the initial plan for that particular problem in the case record.

Each time a problem list is read any user should consider whether the titles of the problems are appropriate, whether they remain 'active' or 'inactive' (*See* Ch. 2), and whether relationships exist between apparently distinct problems. It is also useful to select an active problem, at random, and check the appropriateness of the plans and follow up notes for that problem.

The numbering of problems in a master problem list should not be changed during subsequent contacts with the patient because this breaks the thread of evolution of the problems through the record. Such changes usually occur inadvertently when previous notes are not available at the time of interview, or if a previously constructed problem list has been misfiled in the notes. We have also noted that changes in the numbering of a general practitioner's problem list have been made by hospital doctors. This is unfortunate. Although the numbers should not be changed, there is no limitation on changing or refining the title of the problem (Fig. 3.1). This does not disrupt the continuity of the evolution of the problem in the notes.

The design of the master problem list is not rigid. Some authors recommend the use of lines to allow for changes in the titles of individual problems. It is also helpful to use paper which is more durable than the rest of the case notes. The reverse side of the master problem list may be used to print further spaces for problems, or , as in our maternity hospital, to print a section to record a detailed reproductive history (Fig. 3.15). However, our experience has been that it is useful to record the recommended procedural guidelines of POMR on the reverse side of the problem list (Fig. 3.2). This is of considerable assistance to individuals who are unsure of the system and who may have lost, or who may not have received written instructions on the use of POMR.

We have found that 16 spaces are sufficient for the master problem list for most case records. In our experience the number of problems per patient has ranged from one to 27, with a mean of seven of which four are active. In older patients a second master problem list may be required.

The master problem list should always be filed at the front of the record so that any user of the record can be aware, at a glance, of the principal active problems.

It is inappropriate to take codings for statistical returns from the master problem list because this list does not always represent an order of clinical priority, particularly if repeated admissions are represented on the problem list, or if the list is made up in some chronological order.

The provisional problem list. We have found that it is very helpful to define an area in the notes immediately following on from the physical examination sheet to record provisional (or temporary) problems (Fig. 3.7). We encourage students and house officers to use this list to declare their uncertainties about such findings as cardiac murmurs, ill-defined problems, diagnoses, findings and abnormal biochemical results. Fragmentation of problems also becomes less frequent once students and junior staff gain experience and benefit from constructive comment from more senior staff. As discussed elsewhere (Ch. 2) several symptoms may be considered together, e.g. anorexia, weight loss and vomiting. To make a plan for each separately is obviously

PREVIOUS OBSTETRIC HISTORY

Preg. No.	Date	Place	LABOUR and DELIVERY				INFANT			
			Gest.	Onset sp/ind	Dur Hrs.	Mode of Delivery	Sex	Weight	LB/SB 1st week Death	Name and Unit No.
1	Complications:						Feeding:			
2										
3										
4										
5										
6										
7										

Fig. 3.15 Alternative use of reverse side of problem list shown in Figure 3.1. This is used in the Maternity Hospital.

unsound, cumbersome and a misuse of the system.

An order of clinical priority is used in the medical wards in drawing up the provisional problem list. The list, as mentioned above, *supplements* the master problem list until the discharge summary is written. At that time all provisional problems must be either integrated into other problems, or transferred to the master problem list, or resolved (Fig. 3.7). They must not be lost! As with entries on the master problem list it is essential to record the date of entry of the problem in the record so that cross reference to the follow up notes is facilitated. Note that a letter prefix, e.g. A, B, C distinguishes provisional problems.

In obstetric practice, where patients are often seen in an emergency by staff who are unfamiliar with the case, it has been found to be useful to present the provisional problem list on a cut-out section which is clearly visible whichever part of the case sheet is in use. The cut-out is divided into three sections:

1. Antenatal problems
2. Delivery and post-natal problems
3. Paediatric problems.

Each provisional problem list is used for the duration of the pregnancy and is normally initiated by a consultant at the first outpatient booking consultation. Therefore, in the obstetric notes the order of priority of the provisional problems is chronological, as the list is added to during antenatal care and when the patient is admitted for delivery.

Plans

Several points of detail are worth emphasising.

The plan for the problem relating to the principal presenting complaint should be the *first* entry. Obviously the order of discussion of the plans for each individual problem should follow an order of clinical priority. We do not use separate sheets to record the progress of individual problems. We feel that this is impractical, unrealistic and wasteful of space in the case records.

Some users advocate the use of stationery which is pre-printed with the recommended POMR format for plans. We do not do this because we feel that this is inconvenient, emphasises the format unnecessarily and follow up notes are of variable length. The writing of initial plans is straightforward and has been discussed elsewhere in this book (Ch. 2). A sensible approach is required. It is *not* essential always to record, for *each* individual problem *each* of the plan guideline headings (i.e. Dx, Mx, Rx, Ex). An initial plan might read *3. Smoking Ex.* told to stop! or

2. Social Plan: contact social worker (Fig. 3.7).

We have not been successful in recording goals to aim for in the management of all problems. Many problems are ill-defined and a description of goals is often inappropriate. Nevertheless, goals are stated frequently in follow up notes of problems such as obesity and hypertension or in discharge summaries when the clinical situation is clearer.

In the obstetric case sheet plans are recorded alongside the cut out list of active problems to which they relate. This area is suitable for plans which constitute a definite instruction, eg. repeat elective Caesarean section. If fuller detailed plans are to be written they are recorded in the admission notes in the recommended form.

Follow up notes

It is our experience that misunderstandings are common about this aspect of the POMR system.

The important point to understand is that slavish adherence by clinicians to the entire S.O.A.P. form *each* time an entry is made about an individual problem is *not* obligatory, particularly in acute clinical situations, and in rapidly evolving problems. Indeed, in these situations flow sheets are preferable. The S.O.A.P. guidelines, nevertheless, are a useful prompt to consider for each problem.

1. S — subjective complaints
2. O — objective findings, including laboratory tests
3. A — assessment,
4. P — plans
   a) for diagnosis (Dx)
   b) for monitoring type information (Mx)
   c) for treatment (Rx)
   d) for education of the patient (Ex)

Examples of typical follow up notes are shown elsewhere in this volume. Entries by consultant staff and occasional entries by nurses, usually for social problems, are also in a S.O.A.P.-style format but an occasional overview summary statement by a consultant is also helpful.

Another area of difficulty concerns the recommendation in the POMR system that the recording of *all* results of investigations should come under the Objective part of the S.O.A.P. guidelines. While this is of much value, particularly as an educational aid, we have usually limited the recording of results in relation to specific problems to important and relevant negative or positive results. In our experience the recording of *all* results leads to congestion of the follow-up notes, and the notes become tedious to follow, and use up valuable time and paper. We feel that the principle of recording *all* results is a good one but that it is more relevant to apprentice students than to busy house staff. The filing of laboratory results is discussed later in this chapter.

We have experienced few difficulties with other aspects of the follow-up notes. In particular, users have appreciated the usefulness of clear *numbering* or *lettering*, and *underlining*, of problem titles. Clear headings are of great assistance in following the evolution of specific problems. The broad S.O.A.P. guidelines are also helpful to students who wish to compare their own findings and plans with the plans of the ward team. Flow sheets are not exclusive to POMR and have been used widely.

The POMR may occasionally cause irritation during busy clinics or ward rounds because decisions require to be made about problems which have been defined and about their plans. On the other hand this is useful and instructive and is of benefit to both patient and to users of the record.

Operation notes are entered in a pre-printed part of the case sheet. The problem, say *1. Uterovaginal prolapse* is then further refined on the master problem list to include the procedure, eg. *1. Uterovaginal prolapse* – Manchester repair.

Newcomers to POMR write too many notes until they gain some experience. Verbal padding must be avoided. The record should be efficient and facilitate care, not exhaust the contributor.

Paper is also saved if relevant entries are made across, rather than down, the casesheet pages, i.e. *A. chest pain* S → O → Rx → Ex.

Discharge summary

This is the final follow-up note of an inpatient admission. In whatever form it is completed there should be the minimum delay in sending the summary to the practitioner. We now circulate a list showing *all* summaries outstanding for over two weeks following the patient's discharge from hospital.

We believe that the introduction of the structured problem-orientated summary contributed greatly to our improved in-patient use of POMR. A doctor from each team in the ward is responsible (in rotation) for timely completion of the summary. Ease of completion depends on the standards of supervision and adequacy of the record which are currently prevalent in the ward. Omissions and poor planning in the follow-up notes are readily identified and the reliability, thoroughness, analytical sense and efficiency of the ward team are thus under further continuous assessment and the ward staff are given immediate feedback.

The discharge summary shown in Figures 3.8 and 3.9 was designed after consultation with practitioners in the area. Space is available to record both positive and relevant negative information which has been requested by practitioners. The spacings were allocated after calculation of the optimal requirements for at least 95 per cent of the patients discharged based on serial evaluation of space required in previous structured summaries. Different discharge summaries have been designed for other specialities (Fig. 3.16).

The discharge comment about each active problem is in the form of a follow-up note. We do not use a full S.O.A.P. format but concentrate instead on the assessment and plans for each problem. Comments are made about individual problems *in order of priority* of the problems relevant to the current admission. The problem titles are numbered and underlined as in a follow-up note. The principal presenting complaint must be explained by the first comment on a problem. The order of priority of discussion of problems is helpful to the morbidity section within the records department who base their statistical diagnostic returns on this easily identifiable section of the discharge summary, and *not* on the problem list.

The response of our general practitioner colleagues has been favourable. A survey of 120 local practitioners brought 93 separate anonymous replies. Five questions were asked but not all practitioners answered all questions.

1. 69 doctors (out of 76 replies) agreed, or strongly agreed that the new format was acceptable.
2. 69 doctors (77) agreed, or strongly agreed that the problem list was useful.
3. 70 doctors (80) felt that the brief comments on individual active problems were useful. Some commented on specific plans about individual patients and sought further information.
4. 67 doctors (75) felt that the POMR summary was more useful than the former structured summary.
5. Two doctors were concerned that 'whole patient' medicine might be lost.

Our *out-patient letters* are also written in a problem-orientated form. The problems are numbered, problem titles underlined and, broadly, the S.O.A.P. format is used but without typing *S.O.A.P.* as such. We do not feel that we have lost touch with the family doctor. Literary style and personality need not be dampened by the format. We do not comment on all active problems in each letter but concern ourselves with the clinically important current problems. For example, the letter may include a follow-up note on *7. Hypertension, 8. Psoriasis* and *3.*

Aberdeen Hospitals	PATIENT'S NAME and ADDRESS:		Unit No.
GYNAECOLOGICAL P.O.M.R. Summary Sheet			D. of B.

Occupation			Marital State
Ward		Hospital	Consultant
Date on W.L.		Transferred from	Referred by
Admitted		Discharged	Disposal

G.P.

PRESENTING HISTORY and EXAMINATION

Investigations

Code	Operation

Pathology

Medicines Administered

Adverse Effects

MASTER PROBLEM LIST	No.	
No.		

Code	Diagnoses	Comment (including follow-up recommendations)

S 31
POMR

Fig. 3.16 Discharge summary, gynaecology.

Obesity. The omission of a reference to problems, *1, 2, 4, 5, 6* is a reminder to the practitioner that other problems have been identified in previous correspondence or in discharge summaries.

Users

We have found that the POMR system affects members of the ward team in different ways. Many of these have been discussed elsewhere in this and other chapters.

The *houseman* has clear guidelines to record keeping. He soon learns to declare his uncertainties on the provisional problem list. He also becomes familiar with rational plans for common problems. He comes face to face with his own standard of performance because his actions and plans are closely scrutinised by all team members, and students. Most house officers have regarded the continuous audit and comments from senior staff as helpful and have accepted that their notes were for communal use, and were not inviolate personal writings. They have found that POMR offers a useful aid to training because each problem is dealt with along similar guidelines. Of course some 'individualistic' traditional systems also offer similar benefits.

Our experience has been that our housemen do not feel that POMR notes take longer to write than a good, traditional record, *provided that* with either system they are not responsible for refiling chaotic old notes!

The benefits to *senior staff* have been outlined elsewhere. Our experience is that less time is wasted on ward rounds and at outpatients because the case record should be in order and the evolution of problems should be clear. The POMR system is also helpful to doctors when on call for unfamiliar patients. The section in the follow-up notes which refers to the education of the patient about each problem should also be especially helpful in preventing unnecessary variations in the advice given to patients. *Nursing staff* also appreciate the opportunity to use, and contribute to, the notes. They have said that they felt the lack of POMR when moving to new units. *Secretarial staff* say that the discharge summaries are more interesting to type, and that less typing is involved than with our previous system.

EXTENSION OF POMR IN HOSPITALS

A little picture is worth a million words

– Chinese proverb

If a limited introduction 'pilot scheme' by a team is successful, and a group of individuals understands the limitations and common misuses of POMR, successful gradual extension to other units and hospitals is feasible because the system can be discussed and demonstrated in clinical practice in case notes chosen at random in wards or outpatient clinics. The difficulties of successful extension of POMR should not be underestimated.

We have found that misunderstanding or usually ignorance of the concept and practice of POMR is the commonest cause of resistance to extension of the system. Indeed, our own initial hostility was due to misunderstandings about jargon and inflexibility. In addition, the medical profession tends to be wary of change for the sake of change, and of enthusiasm for things just because they are new. The association of POMR with fragmentation of problems, audit and computers has also led to an element of fear and prejudice which has occasionally precluded a rational choice by potential users between POMR and other traditional recording systems, sometimes before the basic principles (of either!) have been understood. This is unfortunate because, in our view, the system has much to contribute to patient care, and to the education of the users *if it is properly used.*

Some of the advantages and disadvantages of POMR have been discussed elsewhere in this volume. In our own discussions about the advantages and disadvantages of POMR with different individuals the following (rough) personal quotes (unattributed!) have been made —

— 'Unless all change, why bother?'
— 'POMR will collapse in six months'
— 'Burn all records and start afresh each time'
— 'POMR is too obsessional, introverted and analytical. It carries self-analysis to absurd extremes, like spelling out how to walk'
— 'The obvious and accepted dressed up in pseudo-intellectual jargon; ill-placed evangelism'
— 'Of course we know the concepts well already and try to practise them; in a few years it will settle down into a few useful procedural advances'
— 'The index is super, much of the rest is a bit silly'
— 'I'm all for it, after I've retired'
— 'I'm doing it already, I think, sort of . . .'
— 'POMR is about systems, not people'
— 'More time is spent taking care of the notes than taking care of the patient'
— 'My standard of care is jolly good without POMR'

We believe that POMR is an interesting and useful advance in recording and education, *if* it is approached and practised with flexibility, perspective, understanding and temperance.

Successful extension depends, in our experience, on acceptance by the *consultant* of the need for a fair trial of the POMR system. If his goodwill, interest, participation and particularly understanding are added, successful extension should occur. Otherwise as discussed in the section on use and maintenance, the system will collapse and get a bad name, partly due to predictable misuse.

Extension also depends on the motivation of the ward team. Juniors tend to adapt to POMR more quickly than seniors but unless they are interested, and understand the conceptual and practical implications of POMR, we believe that there is no value in forcing them, or attempting to persuade them to change their methods of record keeping. Spoonfeeding or the enthusiasm of one or two individuals cannot sustain the system indefinitely.

It is also important in the early stages of extension, as mentioned earlier, not to draw up battlelines about definitions and procedural details. Discussions are much more informed once potential users have some experience of the system. The reasons for the existence of the procedural guidelines will then be clearer. In addition, the recurring exposure of the individual to his alternative system of note-keeping will provide a contrast which may help him to choose between the 'old' and 'new' systems.

Conversion of records should be gradual. We recommend that a start be made with patients newly admitted to hospital, followed gradually by conversion of all outpatient case notes. Of course, at outpatients it is seldom possible to peruse the entire, often bulky, disordered record within the time available for each consultation. Such notes should be set aside so that the problems can be defined and then discussed with the patient at a subsequent outpatient visit. Not infrequently discharge of the patient from the clinic then results, sometimes after years of follow up for indeterminate reasons. In our experience with some bulky sets of case notes which are not problem-orientated, a review appointment is sometimes made because a real anxiety exists that somewhere in the case notes some important problem or clue lies undetected. This process may be repeated at a subsequent consultation, particularly if another team member, also unsure of the contents of the notes, and also pressed for time, reviews the patient.

The simultaneous practice of POMR and non-POMR recording is a source of difficulty. In the Aberdeen Teaching Hospitals group a 'unit filing' system is used and until recently chaotic, disordered note folders were common. However, a new filing system has been devised recently and introduced widely. The task of refiling the contents of the old folders into a logical sequence is now being carried out by records staff assisted by facilities provided by the Job Creation Scheme. A description of the system, which also permits editing of the case record to microfilm, or destruction, after specified periods of time has been prepared for publication (Wilson *et al* 1978). Until the records staff took over the new rearrangement of the contents of the old case folders our junior staff rearranged the records themselves because they became so frustrated with the disorder present in the old notes. The mixture of two new systems – one of record keeping (POMR), and another of filing (the new Aberdeen record) – both introduced in quick succession, led to some confusion among some uninformed individuals who mistakenly attributed the whole disturbance to the POMR system!

We have not integrated the formal, routine nursing records with the medical notes. Extension has not been attempted because complexities of nurse training programmes, nursing shortages, and rotations of nursing staff have deterred us. Nevertheless, as mentioned earlier, our senior nurses are encouraged to contribute to the follow up notes, when relevant. Some clinicians do not favour this development.

At the time of writing over half of the acute general medicine wards, the geriatric unit, and the wards associated with the Department of Obstetrics and Gynaecology in the Aberdeen Teaching Hospitals group are attempting to follow the principles of POMR with varying degrees of success.

In our own ward we have succeeded in extending the system to use computer facilities. This has been described elsewhere (Lindsey, Meredith and Petrie, 1977). An example of a section of the computer printout is shown in Figure 3.17. Extension of this computer system to other wards and to general practice is in progress.

CONCLUSION

Successful, simultaneous 'across a hospital' introduction of POMR is a major undertaking and we do not believe that this approach will often result in successful widespread implementation of POMR (Fernow *et al* 1977). Extension from a limited introduction by a small group requires contributions from informed and interested individuals who fully understand the uses, misuses and limitations of POMR.

We believe that the POMR system, *used properly*, has advantages over informal or anecdotal systems of case note writing. The benefits, educational and practical, depend on close supervision of the sensible use of the system. Implementation and maintenance of a POMR system in hospitals cannot succeed without a clear understanding of the aims of the system by senior and junior staff and by medical students. However, in our experience, it is the attitude of *senior staff*

```
*****************************
NAMES AND DATA ARE FICTITIOUS
*****************************

General Medicine: Dr A. Clinician                 Woolmanhill  15, 5,78

PATIENT - (Surname)   SMITH                        UNIT NUMBER → 872246
+------                                            -----------
          (Forenames) John    ,

     Birth Date -  5. 7.17 ,now aged 61 years
     Patient is male  , marital status is single

     Permanent home address →     2 Main Street
                                   Aberdeen
                                   AB1 2MS

GENERAL PRACTITIONER             -     Dr.A N Fmdee
+--------------------+                 The Surgery
                                       Aberdeen

PAST HISTORY / MASTER PROBLEM LIST
+---------------------------------+            Please indicate below
Active:                                           AMENDMENTS
     1. (1963) Ischaemic heart disease
        1.1 (1963) Infarction, myocardial
        1.2 (1975) Infarction, myocardial
     2. (   0) Obesity
     4. (1975) Osteoarthritis
     6. (1976) Psoriasis

Inactive:
     3. (1930) Tonsillectomy
     5. (1974) Smoking
                                          ****************************
     NOTE: To add new problems,use space below    * Please rank below*
           Activity  No.  Date    Title          *PROBLEMS DISCUSSED*
A                                                 *                  *
D                                                 *       [  ]       *
D                                                 *       [  ]       *
E                                                 *       [  ]       *
N                                                 *       [  ]       *
D                                                 *       [  ]       *
A                                                 ****************************

LAST CONTACT WITH GENERAL MEDICINE:      5. 2.76 as Out-Patient (see over)
+----------------------------------+
     Problems Discussed →
              1.  Ischaemic heart disease
              4.  Osteoarthritis

     Recommended  Medication →
     Start  Prob.                    Dose    Route  Freq.  Finish (if
     mth/yr  nu.                                           Date  known)
     2/76   1.0   Digoxin           .125mg   Oral   x2
     2/76   1.0   Frusemide          80 mg   Oral   x1      20/ 4/76
     2/76   1.0   Frusemide          40 mg   Oral   x1      20/ 4/76
A
D
D
E
N
D
A
```

Fig. 3.17 Computer 'patient profile' sheet used at outpatients.

which is crucial. Without their support junior staff and medical students cannot maintain a useful system, or derive the benefits.

ACKNOWLEDGEMENTS

We would like to acknowledge the invaluable assistance of all individuals (doctors, nurses, secretarial and records staff) who have contributed to the development and gradual extension of the POMR system in the Aberdeen Teaching Hospitals groups over the last six years. We are also particularly grateful to the following individuals who kindly read and commented on an earlier draft of this chapter: Professor A. S.

Douglas, Dr. N. Edward, Dr. A. W. Johnston, Dr. L. A. Wilson, Dr. R. D. M. Scott, Dr. C. C. Smith, Dr. H. Deans, Dr. A. J. Hedley, Dr. D. C. Moir, Dr. A. K. Scott, Dr. D. Taylor and Mr. K. Ewen. In addition we are grateful to Dr. M. I. K. Berkeley and Mr. F. D. Damodaran of the Grampian Medical Computer Project for their contribution to the early development of the system in our unit.

Dr. H. R. Millar was in receipt of a Junior Fellowship in Community Medicine sponsored by the Scottish Home and Health Department.

REFERENCES

Fernow, L. C., McColl, I., Mackie, C. & Rendall, M. (1977) An analysis of the use of problem oriented medical records (POMR) by medical and surgical house officers: factors affecting use of this format in a teaching hospital. *Medical Education*, 11, 341–346.

Lindsey, D. C., Meredith, A. L. & Petrie, J. C. (1977) An experimental database for clinical and administrative use. Medcomp 77, Berlin, 725–740. *Online conferences*, Uxbridge, England.

Wilson, L. A., Petrie, J. C., Dawson, A. A. & Marron, A. C. (1978) The new Aberdeen medical record. *British Medical Journal*, 2, 414–415.

4

Implementation of problem orientated medical records in general practice

M. G. SHELDON[1] and A. J. TULLOCH[2]

[1] General practitioner, Banbury, Oxon.
[2] General practitioner, Bicester, Oxon; Research assistant, Unit of Clinical Epidemiology, Department of the Regius Professor of Medicine, Oxford University

Much criticism has been levelled at general practice records and most of it is justified. Although a lot of information is recorded, retrieval is usually difficult. Often there are serious omissions (Cormack, 1970). For example, one of us (Tulloch, 1976) studied the records of new patients reaching his practice. In parous women only 22 per cent of the notes contained any record (however modest) of all pregnancies, and in many cases where the pregnancy was recorded the details of care and delivery were incomplete. Only 30 per cent of the women taking the contraceptive pill had any record of this in their notes.

The present conventional record envelope is too small. All notes, letters and results tend to be stuffed haphazardly inside. Progress notes may contain relevant information but may be illegible and unstructured. It is often easier and quicker to take a new history from the patient than to search through the record. Rarely are the notes or letters filed chronologically. Not infrequently the record envelope contains a chaotic mixture of symptoms, findings, investigations, diagnoses of varying certainty, specialist's opinions and general practitioner's guesses. The fact that the record often takes several months to arrive after the patient has registered with a new general practitioner reflects a general lack of concern about the availability of records.

These deficiencies are particularly obvious when a doctor takes over a new practice and finds the records to be inadequate. Necessary information about the patients may have departed with the previous doctor. Clinical decisions are hampered until the new doctor can build up his own 'data base' about the patients. In addition, with the introduction of team care, standards of communication must be improved. More information has to be shared and the medical record is the only sensible place to keep it.

The time is ripe for a general improvement in record keeping. However before instituting any new system we need to consider the special problems of general practice which make good record keeping difficult.

Firstly, the record envelope in use is no longer suited to the needs of primary care (Corbett, 1962, Last, 1966, Acheson, 1967, Hodson, 1967 and Abrams *et al* 1968). It is not a file but an envelope which will not accept commonly used sizes of paper without folding or cutting. The small cards which the practitioner has to write on soon become dog-eared and difficult to read. The contents of the whole envelope often have to be tipped out and shuffled to retrieve the relevant pages. Most hospital letters are A4 or A5 size and when using the Family Practitioner Committee record envelope they have to be removed, unfolded, refolded and reinserted each time they are consulted. This is a powerful disincentive to use of the file, especially during a busy surgery. Nevertheless some doctors do manage to keep excellent records in these circumstances but this is a tribute to their conscientiousness and perseverance rather than a reflection of the suitability of the record envelope.

Secondly, time is at a premium in general practice. Doctors believe that clinical care must come before record care, so that when pressures occur the record suffers. Unfortunately, time is subsequently wasted because adequate information has not been recorded. Most doctors will have experienced the frustration of trying to find out what therapy has been given to a patient because the 'other doctor' did not record it in the notes and the patient has transferred the little white pills to a different container. Time 'saved' by not keeping adequate records is usually 'lost' at a later stage with consequent frustration to the doctor and occasionally grave danger to the patient.

A third problem in general practice is that the doctor knows far more about his own patients than could possibly be entered in the record file. However, this should not be used as an excuse for omission unless the practitioner intends being always on duty and never wishes to delegate to other doctors and ancillary staff.

In addition, the handwriting of doctors is notoriously illegible. The only parts of the record which are invariably readable are the typewritten letters from specialists. Some practices make a habit of typing all or part of their records and this is a great help to others who need to use them in the future.

The nature of conditions encountered in general practice is also different from that found in hospital practice. Most consultations are for minor self-limiting conditions and lengthy notes of these are usually inappropriate. Acute serious illnesses are often referred for specialist advice and the consequent record of events is contained in letters, summaries, discharge notes and continuation sheets so that the story is fragmented and may be difficult to unravel in the future. The records usually lack integration, leave important data inaccessible and do not give a clear profile of the condition.

As if all these difficulties were not enough in themselves, the major stumbling block to any advance in record keeping is the attitude of general practitioners (Dawes, 1972). General practitioners tend to be individualistic even when working in groups and uniformity may be positively resisted. Structuring of records is disliked and the practitioner will often use the records solely for his own convenience. The record is usually viewed as an aide-memoire for future use in clinical situations, and occasionally legal ones. Before any change can be made, doctors will have to accept that shortcomings exist in their records and that it is important to rectify these. If medical audit becomes a feature of general practice in the future, either voluntarily or compulsorily, records will have to improve as they may be needed for audit of clinical care.

Several requirements are necessary to bring about an improvement in the standards of record keeping in general practice. Firstly, all doctors, medical students, nurses and ancillary staff will have to be educated in the values and methods of record keeping. Secondly, some new form of file will have to be adopted to replace the present record envelope. This could be a more appropriate folder size such as A5 or A4 with facilities for filing notes and letters chronologically, or a system making use of modern recording techniques such as microfilm or computers. Many practices are using the A4 size folder which is standard throughout the hospital service, and finding that good record keeping is facilitated by the larger format which allows sensible filing of its contents (Loudon, 1975). However, it must be emphasised that good record keeping relies more on the method of recording than on the size of paper or medium which is being used.

The third requirement for improvement in general practice records is a system of recording which allows easy input and quick retrieval of information by all members of the primary care team. The method of recording learned by medical students in the most hospital wards is quite inappropriate to general practice. Many doctors now maintain that POMR will not only improve hospital records but can also be adapted for use in general practice to improve record keeping significantly (Bjorn and Cross, 1971).

The philosophy and practical implications of problem orientated records satisfy the recording needs of general practice for clinical care, education, audit and research. Keeping such records takes little more time than any other method and will usually save time in the long run by making the information more easily retrievable. The cost of conversion to POMR is minimal and if all members of a practice participate in the exercise, long term benefits will accrue to all who use the record.

DESCRIPTION OF POMR IN GENERAL PRACTICE

The data base

The data base is the term used for the information about a patient which is needed before a doctor can make sensible clinical decisions (*See* Ch. 2). In emergencies it is possible to institute therapy without any background knowledge of the patient, but usually the greater the amount of relevant information available, the more likely are the clinical decisions to be correct.

Knowledge of past illnesses and family predispositions to illness may point the way to the correct diagnosis. Previous allergies or hypersensitivities must be taken into account before prescribing further drug treatments. An awareness of the patient's work and social background will lead to sensible directions for the patient to follow.

Some general practitioners with a good memory carry a sizeable amount of information about many of their patients in their heads. Unfortunately, memories fail, doctors take time off, and a patient may see many different doctors in quite a short space of time.

It is therefore desirable that the important part of this background information should be contained in the patient's record in an easily retrievable form. The data base section of a problem orientated record will consist of a few sheets of E.C.5 card or A4 paper. This can be partly structured to facilitate the entry and retrieval of information.

Even in well kept conventional records, the background information may be scattered in various places in the notes. Some may appear on a summary sheet, other items of information will be found in the letters and continuation sheets, whilst important facts may appear in red ink on the front of the record. Each doctor uses his own system and although he may be familiar with it himself, it is of little use to any other doctor using the record. We therefore strongly recommend that a commonly accepted data base is used in any one practice so that all the information collected is readily available in the same place in the record. Any gaps in the information are then obvious and if the structuring is reasonably uniform, it will be of use to all who need to use the notes.

Defining the data base
Before suitable stationery can be designed the data base must be defined. Groups of practitioners must agree on the acceptable amount of information which should be collected and recorded within the practice. Too much information is often counterproductive as important items may then be lost amongst less important ones. Similarly, too small a data base is of little use as important items may be missing.

Although each doctor may wish to define his own data base much of the information collected will be common to all. However, local variations affect each practice so that the data base collected will reflect the area in which the patient lives and the personal interest of the doctor. For example, doctors in rural areas may wish to include the pets and farm animals with which the patient comes into contact, whilst in an urban area, the doctor may decide to include close proximity to a motorway or area of heavy traffic. It may be important to know a patient's nationality and religion. Thus the data base of a practitioner in the middle of bedsitter land in London will differ from that of a practitioner in the heart of Oxfordshire, but much of the information will be common to both.

The following list contains the information which we think should be collected from every patient in the practice and recorded on suitably designed sheets in the notes.
Essential information in the data base
Name and address.
Date of birth, sex, marital status, nationality.
Occupation and details of work actually performed.
Allergies and hypersensitivities.
Previous illnesses, accidents and operations.
Positive family history for certain inherited illnesses.

Smoking habits.

Obstetric history in women.

Additional information which may be valuable

Social details such as housing, and family ties.

Personal profile of the patient (including hobbies and amount of physical exercise taken).

Immunisation details in children.

Routine physical data e.g. height, weight and blood pressure (in adults).

Other information relevant to the practice as discussed above.

(e.g. pets, religion and local hazards).

Collecting the data base

Data base information should be collected when the patient first registers with a new general practitioner. The receptionist or person accepting the medical cards should collect the information relating to name, address, age, sex, occupation, marital status and nationality. Much of this information is recorded on the front of the medical records when they are received from the Family Practitioner Committee but the records usually take several weeks to arrive, and are often out of date or incorrect. Medical and personal information in the data base should also be obtained when the patient first registers.

There are several ways in which this information can be collected. The usual way is for the doctor to collect it himself by interview when the patient presents for his first consultation. This gives the doctor an opportunity to 'size the patient up' and enables the relationship to get off to a good start as the doctor shows interest in the patient's problems.

Many practices are now reinforcing this technique with the use of questionnaires which may be filled in either by the patient directly or by an ancillary helper. Most patients can understand and complete a short simple questionnaire at home or whilst waiting to see the doctor. If queries arise it is easier for the doctor to answer them at this early stage in the doctor/patient relationship.

It is of course important that the questionnaire is discussed with the patient at a subsequent consultation as something is nearly always omitted, either intentionally or accidentally. By reading through the questionnaire with the patient present, the doctor can fill in the gaps. A complete data base is obtained in only a few minutes of consultation time. We have found that 80 per cent of patients co-operate with questionnaires. In the others an interview technique has to be used (Sheldon, 1976)

Samples of our questionnaires are shown in Figures 4.1 to 4.4. They are not specific to POMR. These have been in use for several years and have been printed for us by a drug company. Separate sheets are used for children, men and women. The whole questionnaire can be filed in the notes prior to completing the data base. We have purposely used a balanced combination of closed and open questions to encourage the patient to write freely. Much can be learned about the patient from the knowledge he has about his past illnesses.

The routine physical data can be collected by a suitable trained ancillary helper or by the doctor in the surgery. It is important not to be too ambitious in data collection as early enthusiasms may wane. The importance of a defined data base is that it should be collected on *every* patient.

When the old case records arrive in the practice from the previous doctor we look for information which we may not have gathered previously. The patient's current history is then compared with recorded findings and a final data base compiled. In both our practices a nurse or secretary completes the data base from the questionnaires and old records. The information is presented to the doctor for checking. In this way an accurate data base is obtained (preferably typed) with minimal expenditure of time and effort by the doctor.

PATIENT QUESTIONNAIRE

This set of questions has been designed to help your new general practitioner get to know you and your medical problems.

All questions will be handled confidentially but if you are concerned about any of them, please leave them blank. Your doctor will be pleased to answer any questions.

It will be appreciated if you can return the completed forms to the surgery as soon as possible or bring them with you when you first visit the doctor.

NAME..Date of birth.....................

CHILDHOOD ILLNESSES.

Please tick those illnesses which you have had, and if possible, give your approximate age:

Mumps.....................	German measles................................
Measles...................	Scarlet Fever................................
Diphtheria................	Rheumatic Fever..............................
Chickenpox................	Childhood Eczema.............................
Asthma....................	Whooping cough...............................

ILLNESSES, OPERATIONS and ACCIDENTS

Please list all serious illnesses, hospital admissions, operations and accidents with dates and as much information as you can remember.

Fig. 4.1 The first page of the patient questionnaire.

page 2

PRESENT MEDICINES

Please list any medicines or tablets you are taking at present, and the illnesses for which you are taking them.

ALLERGIES

Are you allergic or sensitive to any medicines, food, animals etc.

IMMUNISATIONS

Please tick if you have been immunised against the following illnesses, and if possible give the dates of last vaccinations.

Diptheria . . . .   Measles . . . .

Whooping cough . . . .   Smallpox . . . .

Polio . . . .   German measles . . . .

Tetanus . . . .   Tuberculosis . . . .

BLOOD

Do you know what your blood group is? . . . .

Have you ever been a blood donor? . . . .

Have you ever received a blood transfusion? . . . .

SMOKING

Do you smoke now? . . . . . Cigarettes . . . . . Cigars . . . . Pipe . . . .

If you have now stopped smoking:-

When did you stop? . . . .

What was the maximum smoked? . . . .

If you are still smoking:-

How much each day? . . . .

How old were you when you started? . . . . . .

WEIGHT

What is your weight now? . . . .

Have you lost weight recently? . . . .

Have you put on weight recently? . . . .

continued . .

Fig. 4.2 The second page of the patient questionnaire.

FAMILY HISTORY

Do any of your family or close relations have any of the following illnesses or conditions.

	Yes or No	Please give details
Sugar Diabetes		
High Blood Pressure		
Heart Attack		
Stroke		
Epilepsy or Fits		
Asthma		
Skin Disease		
Nervous Disorders		
Allergies		
Congenital Diseases		
Cancer		
Kidney Disease		
Twins		
Other Diseases		

OCCUPATION

What is your occupation?

What does your job actually entail?

What other jobs have you had in the past?

HOBBIES

Please list your hobbies, recreational and sporting activities

PETS

Please list any pets or animals which you keep

Is there any other information you may think helpful, or are there any problems you wish to discuss with the doctor?

WOMEN ONLY - please turn over to last page.

Fig. 4.3 The third page of the patient questionnaire.

page 4

WOMEN ONLY

PERIODS

At what age did your periods start? . . . .

finish . . . . (if relevant)

Are your periods regular? . . . .

Do you use contraceptives:

The Pill

Intra-uterine coil

Diaphragm

Sheath

Other methods

If you use the pill - how long have you been taking it? . . . .

do you get any side-effects? . . . .

Have you had a cervical (cancer) smear? . . . .

What was the date of the last one? . . . .

CHILDREN

Please list all children that you have had

Name	Date of Birth	Difficulties with pregnancy or birth (and birth weight if known)

Have you had any miscarriages? - please give details

end of questionnaire
THANK YOU.

Fig. 4.4 The final page of the patient questionnaire. This page is only given to women over 16 years of age.

Designing the data base

We have designed data sheets suitable for use in A4 or E.C.5 sized records. We have kept in mind the fact that some information alters with time (e.g. address and occupation) whilst in other parts of the data base new information is added at intervals.

DATA BASE SHEET 1

SURNAME	SMART	SEX	F
First names	Mary Ellen	Date of birth	4 5 52
Maiden name	JONES	N.H.S. number	QNPB 312
		Nationality	Nigerian
Blood Group	O Rh Neg	Practice number	R 301942
Allergies and hypersensitivities	? PENICILLIN (rash in 1974)	Registration date	4 9 72

On REGISTRATION		SUBSEQUENT CHANGES (with dates)	
CIVIL STATUS	Single	July 1977 Married	
OCCUPATION	Student	Jan 75 Secretary	July 77 Housewife
ADDRESS	4 High St Sometown	24 St Mary's Rd. Sometown	
Tel. No	49279		

Date left practice   Reason for leaving

Fig. 4.5 Data base Sheet 1. This is filled in by the receptionist who first registers the patient. All the important basic data is entered. It is best to put allergies in red ink.

The first sheet (Fig. 4.5) contains the basic registration data which should be collected by the receptionist when the patient first registers. Space is left for subsequent changes of address, occupation and marital status. Any allergies and hypersensitivities are entered, preferably in red. This sheet is filed in the front of the patient's record as it contains all the information needed to fill in the numerous forms which the NHS requires. When the patient leaves the practice the date and reason for removal can be added, and the sheet photocopied and kept in the practice for future reference. If NCR paper (No Carbon Required) is used a second copy is created. This is filed by date of birth and sex so creating an age/sex index without further effort (Sheldon 1974).

The second sheet (Fig. 4.6) contains the medical information collected from the patient either by means of a questionnaire or at interview. All illnesses, operations, accidents and other important events in the patient's life are entered chronologically. Important

DATA BASE SHEET 2.

NAME   John SMITH   Date of Birth 14.4.36

FAMILY HISTORY   Father died age 47 Coronary thrombosis
                  Grandmother - maturity onset diabetes

PATIENT PROFILE   Heavy mortgage   Insurance salesman.
                  3 children   Plays cricket for Watchfering

	12.4.75	13.2.76	14.5.77	16.6.77			
Smoking habits	20/day	stopped	10/day				
Weight	70 kg		78 kg				
B.P.	130/80		140/90	150/105 →	HYPERTENSION FLOW CHART		

PREVIOUS ILLNESSES, ACCIDENTS and OPERATIONS.

		SOCIAL EVENTS.
1947	Appendicectomy	
1952	# R. Femur (RTA)	
June 56		Married
1957	D. U. diagnosed	
Jul, 58		Father died coronary
Jan 66	Vagotomy and pyloroplasty	
1972	Rodent ulcer R. cheek	
1976		Wife - major for the year

Fig. 4.6 The second sheet of the data base which contains the medical information. Brief details of family history and patient profile are included. If regular measurements of weight or blood pressure are taken they should be transferred to a flow chart.

problems are entered on the problem list.

Space is provided for blood pressure, weight and smoking habits. Additional boxes are available for subsequent alterations in the findings. If regular readings of weight or blood pressure are taken they should be transferred to a flow chart otherwise this sheet will quickly be filled. If the patient has a long and complicated past history it can be continued on a further sheet.

The third sheet (Fig. 4.7) is for women only and contains a chronological list of all events referring to the reproductive organs.

These three data base sheets are kept in the record and updated when new information comes to hand. The sheets may be cyclostyled or printed and if put into all new records (and old ones as well) a satisfactory data base is quickly built up for each patient.

DATA BASE SHEET 3 - WOMEN ONLY

Menstrual, Obstetric and Contraception Flow Chart

NAME *Mary SMITH*   Date of birth   *19. 2. 24*

DATE	EVENTS
1938	*Menarche*
1940	*Dysmenorrhoea D+C*
1944	*Miscarriage at 12 weeks*
14 3 45	*FTND. Julia. Wt 6lb 2oz. No problems*
29 2 47	*Forceps delivery John. Wt. 8lbs 3oz. Mild P.E.T. Delay in second stage.*
1949	*Stillbirth 38 weeks ? due to toxaemia*
	Advised not to have any more children
Aug. 64	*Menorrhagia ? due to fibroids*
Jan 67	*HYSTERECTOMY — Mr Thurogood at St. Bede's (both ovaries retained)*
Feb 73	*Menopausal symptoms*

Fig. 4.7 The last data base sheet for women only. We feel it best to make a chronological record of all events relating to the reproductive organs.

The problem list

The theory and use of problem lists are discussed in Chapter 2. The general practice problem list is essentially the same as that used in hospital practice but there are special difficulties. For example, the problem list in general practice must constantly be updated in a small percentage of patients with a complex history. Indeed the list of problems may become long and complicated if trivial and temporary problems are entered. It is then increasingly difficult for the doctor to pick out those active problems which he should consider at each consultation.

Ideally the practitioner himself should create the problem list. However it can be compiled by suitably trained ancillary workers *provided* the doctor checks the list afterwards. Help by ancillary staff is an important aid to continued successful use of POMR. A degree of obsessional perseverance is required to keep any good records. Other pressures on the GP make it difficult for him to sustain good records without such support. We have found that an intelligent nurse or medical secretary can produce a problem list after a month or so of teaching by example but of course it must be checked by the practitioner.

PROBLEM LIST

NAME: Julia Jones   Date of birth:

DATE	No.	ACTIVE	INACTIVE
Jan. 75	1	Husband is shift worker	
" "	2	Poor housing ──────────────→	Sept. 76 moved to council house
" "	3	Heavy smoker	
Apr. 75	4	Allergic rhinitis (tree pollens)	
June 75	5	Epigastric pain ──────────────→	Cholecystectomy Feb. 76
		2. 12.75 gallstones on cholecystogram	
July 76	6	Reactive depression	
		Marital problems	
Aug. 76	7	Oral contraceptive first prescribed ──→	Husband vasectomy Feb. 77
Jan. 77	8	Mother just died of ca. breast aged 52 years	

Fig. 4.8 Problem List. If required extra columns can be added to indicate the last date on which the information was updated if this is done by ancillary staff.

Problem list sheets can be cyclostyled or printed to the doctor's requirements. The example shown (Fig. 4.8) is simple. Additional columns may be added to record updating and coding if required. If a member of the ancillary staff is preparing the problem list it is fairly easy to type it at the same time. This increases its usefulness to other doctors.

The problem list must be filed in a prominent place in the record so that it is visible at each consultation. Hidden information is useless information.

The amount of work involved in creating a problem orientated record to this stage should not be underestimated. Using a patient filled questionnaire and the old records it takes on average 10 minutes for a trained person to create the data base and problem list. (This is less than might be expected because many files (especially of children) contain few entries.) If this is compiled by anyone other than the practitioner a further 5 minutes needs to be set aside by the practitioner for the essential process of checking. Any doctor wishing to convert records to POMR must plan carefully in advance otherwise the additional workload at the outset will defeat him.

Progress notes

This is the only part of the conventional general practice record file which is invariably present, but the mixture of often illegible handwriting and ill assorted notes may make them virtually useless to all except the doctor concerned (and even then, many find difficulty in reading their own handwriting).

There are many aids for keeping good progress notes and the four most commonly used are:

1. Coloured inks and pencils to highlight important points. The same effect can be produced by the use of block capitals or boxing important information.
2. Use of diagrams to present physical findings and investigations.
3. Arranging information in columns so that certain items stand out (e.g. putting all drug treatments on the far right hand side of the page).
4. Typing the record.

All of these can be used to advantage whatever record system is used. The introduction of some structuring can improve the usefulness of records still further. The S.O.A.P. formula referred to in Chapters 2 and 3 has been used in different guises in general practice recording for many years. The subjective part of the record is the history and may be divided up into complaints, direct questioning, past history, etc. The objective findings are usually indicated by some sort of symbol (e.g. o/e or O) and the Assessment in the past has been indicated by a differential diagnosis sign $\triangle$. Plans are frequently omitted from the record, but are of great importance if the doctor is going to chart the progress of the patient's illness in chronic disorders. The S.O.A.P. formula for each active problem is a simple way of representing these different parts of the progress notes and aids reference to the notes in the future. In our own practices we do not write a formal 'Initial Plan' entry for each problem. Instead we use the S.O.A.P. structure from the outset.

3.4.77	Headaches and cough. Rx. Actifed co. linctus
7.4.77	Breathlessness on exertion, chronic cough for 3/12. Little or no sputum. o/e chest n.a.d. P.R. 74 reg. No C.C.F. I think he has asthma. Do C.X.R. Spirometry, W.B.C. Rx. Ventolin syrup 10 ml. t.d.s. See 1/52.
14.4.77	Asthma: much better on Ventolin. C.X.R. n.a.d. Spirometry confirms diagnosis. W.B.C. eosinophilia NOTE. Extreme caution if steroids are ever needed because of ? T.B. in 1948. ct Ventolin.
21.4.77	D. & V. Rx. Mist K. et M.
13.5.77	Asthma continues well on Ventolin. No breath- lessness. Having headaches and dizziness ? cause.
24.5.77	Still having headaches ? due to Ventolin. Stop and see what happens.
4.6.77	Now better, avoid Ventolin in future.

Fig. 4.9 Sample page of progress notes with no attempt at structuring or highlighting the information.

Figure 4.9 shows a typical page of a GP's progress notes written in conventional form. This is typed to make it easier to read but it is still difficult to extract the important information quickly. Figure 4.10 contains the same information set out in a structured format with the addition of problem headings, but without problem numbers – which we do not enter.

In the example shown it is easy to pick out each episode and the action taken by the doctor. Important findings are more likely to be seen and acted upon in the future when the present events have long been forgotten. The important problems such as *asthma* and *headaches on taking Ventolin* (salbutamol) would be transferred to the problem list, but the minor self-limiting conditions such as, cough, diarrhoea and vomiting, would not be entered in the problem list unless' they were recurring problems or related to other more important ones.

3. 4. 77		Headaches and cough Rx.actifed co.linctus
7. 4. 77	S	Wheezing and Breathlessness Breathlessness on exertion
		Chronic cough for 2/12 Little or no sputum
	O	Chest n.a.d. P.R. 74 reg. No C.C.F.
	A	ASTHMA
	P	W.B.C., Spirometry.CXR Rx. Ventolin syrup
		See 1/52
14. 4. 77		Asthma
	S	Much better on Ventolin
	O	CXR normal W.B.C. eosinophils Spirometry confirms asthma
		NOTE
		Extreme caution if STEROIDS
		are needed because of ? T.B.
		in 1948
	P	Rx. Ventolin syrup
21. 4. 77		D. & V. Rx. Mist.K.et M.
13. 5. 77		Asthma
	S	Well on Ventolin No breathlessness
		Headache and Dizziness
		? cause
24. 5. 77		Headaches
	S	Persisting ? due to Ventolin Stop Ventolin
4. 6. 77		Headaches on taking Ventolin
	S	Now better
	P	Avoid Ventolin in future

Fig. 4.10 Sample page of structured progress notes following the POMR guidelines. No extra information is included but the important facts are more easily retrievable than in the example in Fig. 4.9.

Flow sheets

In any complicated series of events and especially in a chronic disorder, it is useful to employ a flow chart. This is no less true in general practice where patients with chronic disease will be followed up repeatedly over many years. It is always easy in such cases to forget investigations or examinations because they only need to be checked infrequently (e.g. an ECG in hypertension). The management of every chronic illness in general practice can be improved and made easier by graphic or tabular presentation of the data. Repeated findings are then brought together so that comparisons can easily be made and trends observed. Very few people would consider looking at a list of temperature recordings in preference to a graphic representation. The maternity co-operation card is a well tried method of presenting information in the form of a tabular flow chart to ease ante-natal care. Such charts are especially useful where the patient is seen by different doctors or where numerous other consultations also occur which would confuse any underlying pattern.

MEDICATION RECORD

NAME: Joan STOKES   ADDRESS:

Date started	No	DRUG	DOSAGE	AMOUNT	NOTES
14. 3. 72	1	AMYTAL tabs	15mg. t.ds.	90	for palpitations
19. 5. 76	2	ALDOMET tabs	250mg. t.d.s	90	→ changed to No 4.
19. 5. 76	3	NAVIDREX K tabs	i daily	30	
24.10.76	4	ALDOMET tabs	500mg. b.d.	60	
15. 9. 77	5	LIBRIUM caps	10mg. b.d.	60	
	6				
	7				
	8				
	9				
	10				
	11				
	12				

REPEAT PRESCRIPTIONS   (1/12 supply unless otherwise indicated)

Date		Date	
14. 6. 76	1 + 2 + 3		
29. 7. 76	2 + 3 (2 months)		
14. 10. 76	1 + 2 + 3		
24. 10. 76	4		
16. 12. 76	3 + 4		
1. 2. 77	3 + 4		
4. 3. 77.	3 + 4		
9. 6. 77.	3 + 4		
10. 7. 77.	3 + 4		
11. 8. 77.	3 + 4		
15. 9. 77.	3 + 4 + 5		

Fig. 4.11 A flow chart showing repeat prescriptions for chronic medications. Extra columns can be added to record date of last consultation and period before next consultation is due.

Many practices now use repeat prescription forms and these are further examples of flow charts which most GP's are already familar with. (Other examples of flow charts in use in general practice are contraceptive cards and child development charts). An example of a repeat prescription flow chart is shown in Figure 4.11. This chart helps to prevents errors in the issue of repeat prescriptions, without a consultation taking place. It also enables the doctor to review the frequency of these prescriptions which gives a measure (in most cases) of the patient's adherence to the treatment advised.

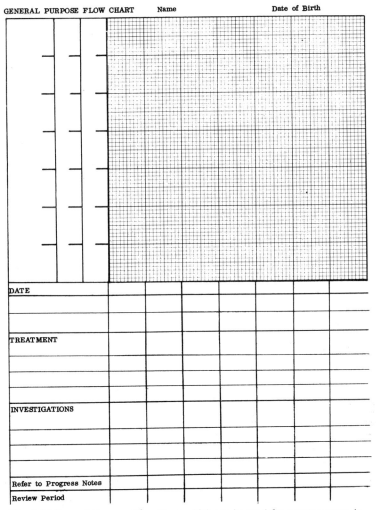

Fig. 4.12 General Purpose Flow Chart which can be used for most purposes in general practice.

The chronic illnesses most usefully represented by means of flow charts are diabetes, obesity, hypertension conditions requiring anti-coagulant therapy, congestive cardiac failure, thyroid disease, asthma, anaemia and other chronic metabolic or hormonal problems.

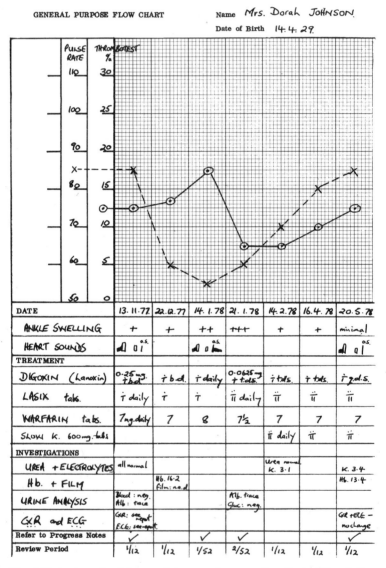

Fig. 4.13 An example of the use of the general purpose flow chart. Although it looks complicated all of the important facts are recorded and progress can be more easily followed.

We have designed a basic chart which can be used in all of the above-mentioned chronic illnesses where the practitioner himself fills in the information (Fig. 4.12). On this chart there is a graphic section with 3 sections which can be used for blood pressure, weight, pulse rate, thrombotest results, blood sugar etc. The rest of the chart is divided to allow space for clinical findings, treatments and investigations. At the bottom is a space for indicating the review period and whether other notes have been entered on the continuation card in the records. This sheet may be printed or photocopied and should prove adequate for most needs. Figure 4.13 shows the chart as used for a patient with mitral stenosis and atrial fibrillation due to rheumatic heart disease being treated with digoxin, diuretics and anti-coagulants. Seven consultations can be represented on the one sheet, but continuation charts can be added without difficulty.

A flow chart specially designed for use in hypertensives by one of us (AJT) is described in Appendix A.

THE USES OF PROBLEM ORIENTATED RECORDS IN GENERAL PRACTICE

The areas of application of any record, including POMR can be classified as follows:

1. Clinical care.
2. Prophylaxis.
3. Education.
4. Record linkage.
5. Research.
6. Report making.

Clinical care

In the clinical situation the GP attempts to gather as much pertinent information as possible about the presenting problem and the previous medical history. Physical examination is then performed, investigations instituted and where possible, a diagnosis made. Finally a decision is taken as to the best way to manage the problem. At most of these stages problem orientation has a contribution to make, and this is particularly so in general practice where time for consultation is generally more limited than in hospital and rapid access to relevant information is particularly important.

The advantages of the problem orientated system have been detailed in previous chapters. It will be recalled that stress is laid on accurate and complete assembly of pertinent data which is well collated and easily retrievable with the logic and objectives of patient management manifest in the records.

As a result of these factors we believe that the doctor, using POMR, enjoys the following advantages in the clinical situation:

1. The full previous medical history is quickly available and helps to direct questions which seek to elucidate the current problem.
2. The structured format of problem list and progress notes enables rapid review of the records and easy access to pertinent information.
3. The fact that the records are well integrated exposes the underlying pattern of the problem, its evolution and response to treatment.
4. The simple descriptive terms which can be used in a problem list make understanding and analysis of the presenting condition easier than if more conventional diagnostic terminology is used. When several problems are involved it is easier to establish priorities which facilitates decision making.
5. Management of the patient can be improved through easier access to pertinent information – for example, the decision to prescribe a particular drug should take into account previous notes on sensitivity, contra-indications or incompatibility – information which is easily available with POMR.
6. The 'patient profile' completes the clinical picture. It may draw attention to previously unsuspected factors, e.g. loneliness in the elderly, and is of particular value in selected groups such as the elderly, the handicapped and the chronic sick.

In addition, although not an integral part of POMR, flow charts have been developed in association with the system and have a fundamental role in the integration of data so that the record file can spell out its message clearly in complex chronic disorders. Their use has been discussed earlier in this chapter and in Chapter 2.

The clinician is thus able to review the presenting problems in the context of the previous history of medical and para-medical disorders affecting health. It is a reasonable assumption that as a result he will be more likely to make an accurate assessment of the situation and institute appropriate measures than if he were less adequately informed. In our experience the more complicated the clinical picture the greater is the value of POMR.

One cannot conclude an appraisal of the value of problem orientation in clinical care without commenting on the effect it has on the doctor's approach to clinical problems in general. The conventional approach lays great emphasis on the importance of making an early diagnosis. This is praiseworthy but it does tend to imply that clinical syndromes are either black or white, whereas in general practice they are all too often grey. Naturally a firm diagnosis should be made when the evidence justifies it, but prior to this stage problem orientation helps in defining vague or complex problems and arranging them in order of priority. It also discourages the doctor from the practice of ignoring or discarding positive clinical findings which cannot be explained. General practitioners are as guilty of diagnostic oversight or error as other doctors. We think that this is less likely using the problem orientated approach with its emphasis on recording problems at the level of understanding of the clinician and the careful integration and tabulation of such data.

Prophylaxis
The emphasis of family medicine is moving towards pre-emptive care with the objective of health maintenance. This involves some form of population monitoring. 'Blanket' screening is now largely discredited (*Screening in Medical Care, 1968*), and case finding during routine consultation and surveillance of 'at risk' groups seem the approaches most likely to be adopted. This involves the identification of patients whose health status is especially vulnerable because of adverse factors which may be medical, social, functional, occupational or economic. Examples of these hazards are as follows:

1. Chronic medical disorders prone to complication e.g. hypertension or obesity.
2. A history of familial disease.
3. Physical handicaps.
4. Major social problems e.g. recent bereavement, an unreliable breadwinner and juvenile delinquency.
5. Occupational disorders, e.g. farmer's lung.
6. Patients defaulting on prophylactic programmes.
7. Patients on multiple or long term therapy.
8. Neonates with adverse pre-natal factors, e.g. placental insufficiency.
9. Elderly patients with multiple problems.
10. Patients with clear evidence of social inadequacy e.g. drug addicts and 'drop outs'.

This list is not comprehensive, but gives some indication of the main areas of special need which should attract more medical and social resources. These resources are unlikely in the foreseeable future to be adequate to deal with the many diverse problems involved. As a result priorities must be established. To do this the patients concerned must be identified, and the needs generated by their disabilities scaled for severity so that medical care can be made available in the first instance where the need is the greatest. To do this a well designed records system is essential in which there is comprehensive assembly of pertinent information in a format which allows easy access to the most important and relevant data (i.e. a defined data base). The information should be well laid out with the objectives of care clearly identified so that the success of treatment can be satisfactorily reviewed. The problem orientated record system meets these requirements.

Of course, much can be achieved using some conventional unsystematised record system, but the existence of shortcomings must be acknowledged. The size and format of many general practice records tends to emphasise the view held by most doctors that the conventional system is simply intended to act as an *aide memoire* for current and occasionally future clinical care for the individual doctor making the records. The scanty haphazard records kept by most family doctors using this system, as documented by Cormack (1970) and Tulloch (1976), serves to emphasise that few doctors see their notes as a source of reference for other doctors or nurses.

The absence of an index and the lack of structure in their system make it clear that record retrieval is not under consideration and, without this, prophylaxis is very difficult to implement. Conventional records can be used to assemble registers of 'at risk' patients, but when the doctor makes no attempt to systematise his records he is unlikely to recognise their value for efficient record retrieval and register assembly in the interests of prophylaxis.

Because of the haphazard data collection the doctor is more likely to be ignorant of health related problems or more prone to overlook them due to the poor access provided by unstructured records without an index.

We believe that doctors using a carefully designed record system such as POMR are more likely to see its value not only as a source of reference in clinical care, but also as a vital tool in prophylaxis. They are, less likely to miss important factors or ignore undefined clinical problems. Review of progress and response to treatment is easier to monitor. Finally doctors and their staff are more likely to be interested in prophylaxis and health maintenance in addition to disease management.

It has long been recognised that demand does not reflect the need for medical care in the community (Last, 1963). The time has surely come for the development and evaluation of screening and surveillance programmes to identify undetected health problems and their complications in the community so that an efficient programme of preventive care can be established. There are three phases of this prophylaxis:

1. Primary – which is concerned with preventing the occurrence of

disease, for example by identifying 'at risk' patients.

2. Secondary – which serves to control the progress of early disease.

3. Tertiary – which relates to the prevention of complications or deterioration of the established disorder and the development of resultant disability.

POMR can play a role in each of these stages. In particular the identification of the patients at special risk is valuable in the primary stage whilst the use of flow charts facilitates review in the other two phases. POMR also encourages both the doctor and the patient to take an interest in health education and health maintenance by stressing the importance of a *comprehensive* collection of pertinent information.

Finally, POMR helps to facilitate the administration of immunisation and other prophylactic programmes since it can improve retrievability of information.

Education

The educational aspects of POMR are discussed in detail in Chapter 5. In general practice certain points deserve fuller discussion.

Conventional undergraduate clinical teaching imbues the student with the importance of collecting information, examining the patient, making a diagnosis and instituting the treatment appropriate to the disorder. Findings which are marginally abnormal tend to be ignored while the clearly abnormal findings which cannot be explained are recorded without special emphasis and then, all too often, conveniently forgotten. In addition, the role of para-medical findings, (e.g. social, functional, occupation, and economic factors) often tend to be underrated as is any information not generated by the doctor himself.

Medical practice calls for a much broader canvas than this and nowhere is this more clearly demonstrated than in family medicine. For example in the case of the elderly and the handicapped the social and economic factors may prove more important for health than the medical disorders. The trainee family doctor must realise this. POMR helps him to do this in the following ways:

1. By laying stress on the value of the comprehensive assembly of pertinent data from all members of the health team (social workers, relatives, etc.).

2. By substituting the flexible classification of problems for the more rigid conventional taxonomy of disease.

3. By encouraging him to record problems at the level of his own understanding.

4. By making him take account of all the health-related problems involved, estimate their relative significance and formulate priorities in care.
5. Lastly by stressing the value of easy access to important information both in the index, and in the structured progress notes to reveal more clearly the underlying clinical message.

The process of *teaching* is also facilitated because the information is carefully organised and therefore easy to interpret by the teacher or the trainee. A good example in clinical approach and recording method can be set, and evaluation of response to the teaching programme facilitated. Thus teaching methods can be made both more efficient and effective.

In essence, the value of problem orientation in teaching is that the records spell out their message clearly, whether it concerns the nature of the clinical care given, the clinical progress, the response to treatment, or the effectiveness of good recording.

In addition when an information system is comprehensive and affords access to pertinent data while reflecting at the same time the logic and objectives of the doctor's approach to clinical care, *audit* is clearly facilitated. The need for some quality control to improve efficiency and effectiveness in the National Health Service is recognised (*British Medical Journal*, 1976). The review of most conventional records is, all too often, an unrewarding exercise since, as Weed (1969) has pointed out, the recorder is playing a game without rules. No standards or criteria have been set, and the rationale of treatment is rarely clear. Record review for the purpose of audit is easier with a problem orientated system.

Record linkage

A system of linked health records brings together selected data of biological interest for a whole population commencing with conception and ending in death, in a series of personal cumulative files, the files being organised so that they can be assembled in family groups. The term record linkage may apply specially to the techniques of assembling the files in spite of errors and omissions in the identifying particulars, or may be used in a more general sense to apply to the organisation involved. (Acheson, 1967).

Clearly the linkage of records from a variety of different sources is easier if the format, system and language of these record files is the same. No other record system offers the degree of uniformity available to those using POMR, with clear guidelines being laid down so that integration of information is much easier.

Research

The classical approach to research is to use the controlled experiment which is carefully planned in advance to test specific hypotheses. For this purpose standardised data are essential. However, as Acheson (1967) has pointed out this approach is suitable only for the analysis of relatively short term conditions, whereas the major problems of the day – chronic and hereditary disease – are longer term problems, never likely to be resolved by the experimental (Hunterian) approach. To complete the picture therefore an alternative, observational (Baconian) approach must also be considered in which data recorded in the course of ordinary clinical care is used to provide experiments. These are after all the records which provide us with statistics, epidemiology, demographic data, aetiology, natural history and prognosis. Such information when recorded in a structured and standardised format such as POMR is more easily retrieved than when conventional recording methods are used.

Report making

The value of carefully laid out and detailed records when reporting to such agencies as the police, solicitors or insurance companies cannot be over-emphasised.

Reporting to and from hospitals can also be made much more effective with POMR. With the latter the patient's current problem is reported in the context of previous disorders. This tends to give a clearer picture of the patient's health status and its evolution as the file accumulates (Tulloch, 1976).

The firmness of the reporting doctor's assessment is generally more obvious than with conventional reports since problems are defined at the level of understanding of the doctor.

The structuring of such reports also makes them more easy to interpret and action requested by the hospital is less likely to be overlooked.

PROBLEMS IN THE USE OF POMR IN GENERAL PRACTICE

An awareness of the problems likely to arise when converting to problem orientated records is essential. Time spent in planning the changeover is never wasted and a regular review of the difficulties encountered is recommended.

The major difficulties encountered in our practices and raised by other doctors may be classified as follows:

1. Problems of attitude.
2. Administrative problems.
3. Lack of objective evidence of the value of POMR.
4. Pre-occupation with the rules of POMR.
5. Cost in time and money.
6. Updating the record.
7. Problems of the abstraction of important information from reports.

Problems of attitude

The difficulties inherent in the introduction and maintenance of a radical new record system are easily underestimated in general practice, as elsewhere.

It is never an easy task to persuade doctors and nurses to change the habits of a lifetime especially in a field like records which they generally regard as peripheral rather than central to their main work, as mentioned earlier in this chapter. Because of poor education in the applications and value of records they accord a low priority to this subject and it is frequently hard to convince them that a sophisticated system such as POMR is necessary in a busy practice. In addition, doctors have been taught to think almost exclusively in terms of tactical (i.e. clinical) care. The strategy of their practice is centred on the need to meet the *demand* for medical care rather than seeking to identify the areas of greatest need. The importance of providing motivation and discipline in the use of this recording system by the advance development of a carefully organised training programme is paramount.

Staff who are unwilling or unable to conform with a standardised approach to recording, such as the structuring of entries in the progress notes, create many difficulties.

New record systems also tend to be associated with computers. These are viewed with suspicion by many doctors and their staff.

Administrative problems

Practical difficulties relating to the time of conversion to POMR and its maintenance have been referred to earlier in this chapter and in Chapter 3. Obviously, a major difficulty can be created if a problem list does not reflect the patient's health status owing to inadequate record assembly, poor problem formulation, unsatisfactory updating and absence of audit. In addition if the extra work-load is allowed to get out of hand it becomes burdensome especially where the health team is already heavily committed. Morale then suffers especially when advance education and motivation have not been provided. Standards are lowered and the risk of a breakdown of the system is increased.

Another problem is the difficulty of ensuring careful recording of relevant information. This does not come easily to most people.

Records of international size A4 lend themselves best to the POMR systems but the conventional, old fashioned FPC records do not preclude its adoption (Tait & Stevens, 1973). The lack of space in the conventional system, however, tends to restrict the use of flow charts and few people developing a POMR system who have also experimented with A4 records want to return to the current FPC record envelope.

Lack of objective evidence of the value of POMR

There is at present little scientific evidence of the value of POMR. One of the authors (Tulloch, 1976) has compared his system with the conventional system and demonstrated its clearcut superiority. 400 consecutive files reaching the practice in Family Practitioner Committee record envelopes were reviewed with the following objectives:

1. To measure the effectiveness of the file in achieving complete assembly of important and pertinent information to which easy access is provided.
2. To estimate the significance of missing information. This exercise was then repeated in 400 files matched for age and sex, housed in files of international size A4 and converted to POMR.

Among incoming files, 77 health-related problems were missing, compared with none in the A4 POMR files. Only factors of significant importance to health were included such as hepatitis, asthma, thyrotoxicosis, open heart surgery etc., ignorance of which had important implications for the clinician. Likewise access was significantly better in the A4 POMR files than in the incoming files because there was an index or problem list, chronological arrangement of the file contents, structuring of progress notes, presence of a treatment chart in chronic disorders, presence of a record of all pregnancies, and details as to whether the patient was taking an oral contraceptive. Finally, the efficiency of the record files was measured by estimating the time taken to identify certain important marker items, and again, except in files with very few entries, the A4 POMR files were more efficient.

The findings of this study confirmed the impression that the POMR system used in one of our practices in the hands of four doctors, *not all of them dedicated to problem orientation*, was appreciably more effective in providing a comprehensive source of relevant information in an easily accessible form and more efficient in yielding such information quickly when used as a source of reference.

Pre-occupation with the rules of POMR

Although problem orientation is more a philosophy than a simple set of rules, many people become bogged down by the procedural details instead of concentrating on the objectives of the system (*See* Ch. 2 and 3). For example the S.O.A.P. formula for progress notes is meant as a guide to the doctor. Usually entries under each heading will not be necessary. With many minor self-limiting conditions it is often not necessary to enter anything in the record except the problem heading and action taken, e.g.:

30.7.77 *Wart on L. hand*   Rx. Podophyllin ointment
14.8.77 *Sprained R. ankle*   Advice on rest and bandaging

The reader will notice that in these examples we have only used the Assessment (for problem heading) and the Plan (for the action taken).

Cost in time and money

The extra costs involved in the use of POMR must be considered. If ancillary staff are used to assist in the keeping of the records then their time must be paid for. Extra sheets will need to be cyclostyled or printed for the data base although existing stationery can be adapted by either the doctor or his staff.   If we assume that each record will take an average of 10 minutes to convert to POMR and the average doctor's list is 2400 patients, then the total conversion time of all the notes to POMR will be 400 hours. Then if approximately 10 per cent of the population leave and are replaced by new patients each year this means an extra 40 hours work per year converting their records. This situation is unique to general practice where the patient may arrive in the practice with an ill-assorted jumble of progress notes and reports often illegibly written and needing to be sorted and sifted.

The updating of records also takes time and approximately 2 hours per week will be needed, although this can usually be fitted into the odd wasted minutes during the surgery sessions.

Updating the record

It is important that records are kept up to date by all who use the record, as an out of date data base, problem list or flow chart may be misleading. It is best at the outset to put the onus of updating on the doctor so that it is done during or at the end of each consulting session by the doctor or by a specially trained member of his staff. It is also advisable for the ancillary staff to check that this has been done from time to time so creating a within practice audit.

Problems of the abstraction of important information from reports

Some doctors prefer to extract the relevant information from letters and laboratory results and enter them under the appropriate problem heading. Others prefer to file hospital letters chronologically, underlining the important sentences. Whichever method is chosen the important problems must be entered on the problem list.

PROCEDURES TO BE FOLLOWED BEFORE INSTITUTING POMR

The problems referred to in the previous section need to be fully appreciated and their implications for the introduction and running of a POMR system fully understood, otherwise major difficulties will arise.

Before starting to problem orientate your records, it is essential to provide motivation. This can only be done by educating the members of the health team in the principles and techniques of the system. Its application in patient care must be clearly described and the benefits which accrue clearly defined. Staff unconvinced of the need for POMR are unlikely to achieve acceptable standards of recording. This will almost certainly lead to breakdown of the system. This applies especially to the doctors, who collect the majority of the information in the data base.

When the motivation for the conversion to POMR has been created the phase of advance planning is reached.

Consideration of the following items is required:

1. Staff members must agree on the amount of information to be recorded.
2. The design of the problem list and the rules for formulation of problems must be agreed i.e. what is to go into the problem list, who is to compile it and who is responsible for audit.
3. The promotion of as much standardisation as is possible among a group of people as individualistic as doctors. It is vital to agree on such issues as the numbering of problems in the records. One doctor failing to do this can cause difficulties.
4. It must be absolutely clear how much of the updating of the record must be done by the doctor and how much can be delegated to other staff. It is extremely important that ancillary staff are briefed carefully about the amount of updating which is to be undertaken.
5. Agreement should be reached on whether to use A4 files or FPC cards.

The final stage in the conversion is the introduction of the new system and this is best done gradually so that staff have time to become accustomed to the changes involved and the new standards of recording expected of them. Problems need to be identified early and dealt with promptly especially where additional workload and cost is concerned. That there will be additional work in the initial stages is inevitable.

Additional recordings must be kept to a minimum as there is a critical point beyond which further recording is counterproductive. Staff should also be warned that, while the procedural guidelines of POMR must be observed, their primary pre-occupation must always be with care of the individual patient.

We have tried in this chapter to outline what we consider to be the most suitable applications of problem orientated records to general practice. We have also attempted to warn about some of the dangers and pitfalls. We hope that this will not deter anyone from using these records as we have found that they consistently improve consultations, minimise mistakes and are simple and easy to use.

APPENDIX A

Hypertension flow chart for general practice (Fig. A.1)
This flow chart has been designed and tested in general practice for use in hypertensives on drug therapy.

On the front of the sheet identifying data, history and physical findings are laid out in a structured format. There are also sections for assessment of the problem and objectives of management. On the reverse side (Fig. A.2) blood pressure and weight recordings are laid out graphically whilst other clinical criteria of progress are set out in tabular form. Finally, there are sections for treatment and the interval before the next appointment. It should be noted that this chart is designed to supplement and not to replace progress notes. Careful cross-referencing with the progress notes is essential when more lengthy records need to be made in the progress notes to amplify the flow charts so that a valid picture of the course of the condition is given. This does not imply reduplication of records.

The objectives of the flow chart are as follows:

1. To assemble and collate all the relevant data at one point rather than leaving it scattered throughout the progress notes.
2. To set out the information in such a manner as to reveal the overall pattern and progress of the disease.
3. To identify clearly the objectives of the treatment, e.g. the

level of systolic and diastolic blood pressure, one is seeking to achieve.

4. To integrate the criteria of review of the hypertension so that a clear profile is given of the disease and its response to treatment. Thus it is possible for the doctor to see clearly whether the objectives of management (e.g. the target diastolic blood pressure) are being achieved.

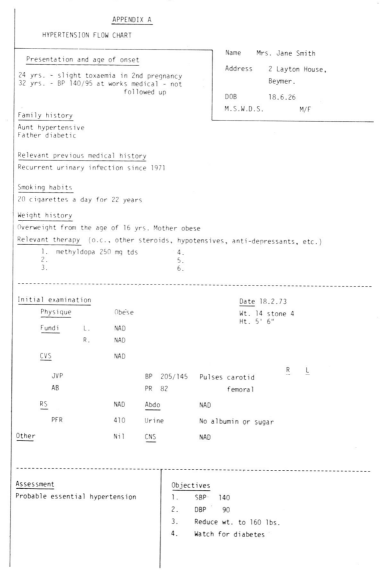

APPENDIX A

HYPERTENSION FLOW CHART

Presentation and age of onset

24 yrs. - slight toxaemia in 2nd pregnancy
32 yrs. - BP 140/95 at works medical - not
                                      followed up

Name   Mrs. Jane Smith

Address   2 Layton House,
                    Beymer.

DOB   18.6.26

M.S.W.D.S.   M/F

Family history

Aunt hypertensive
Father diabetic

Relevant previous medical history

Recurrent urinary infection since 1971

Smoking habits

20 cigarettes a day for 22 years

Weight history

Overweight from the age of 16 yrs. Mother obese

Relevant therapy (o.c., other steroids, hypotensives, anti-depressants, etc.)
        1.   methyldopa 250 mg tds   4.
        2.   5.
        3.   6.

Initial examination   Date 18.2.73

        Physique   Obese   Wt. 14 stone 4
                                             Ht. 5' 6"
        Fundi   L.   NAD

                   R.   NAD

        CVS   NAD
                                                         R   L
           JVP   BP   205/145 Pulses carotid

           AB   PR   82   femoral

        RS   NAD   Abdo   NAD

           PFR   410   Urine   No albumin or sugar

Other   Nil   CNS   NAD

Assessment

Probable essential hypertension

Objectives
1.   SBP   140
2.   DBP   90
3.   Reduce wt. to 160 lbs.
4.   Watch for diabetes

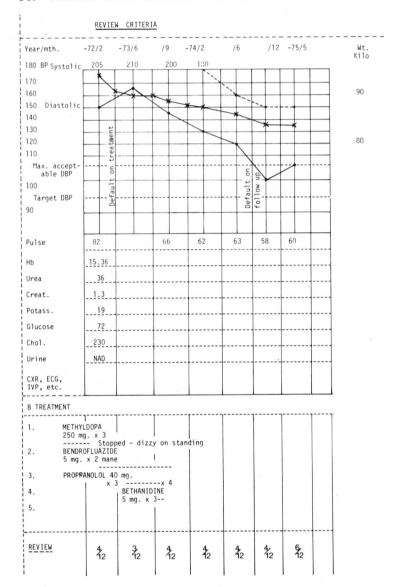

5. To register the drug treatment which the patient is already taking so that incompatibilities are avoided.
6. To emphasise the side effects of treatment already recognised and thus avoid the use of inappropriate therapy in future.
7. To draw attention to other important factors in the

management of the condition such as the patient's adherence to recommended treatment, the regularity of his attendance for review, and associated medical disorders, e.g. myocardial infarct.

8. To form a check list of review criteria and to remind the doctor when these were last checked.
9. To facilitate audit and research by improving record retrieval.
10. To provide a tool for teaching the review of chronic disease.

As a result of all these factors review of the hypertension is greatly facilitated especially if the doctor is not familiar with the patient. Thus in the example shown a doctor unfamiliar with Mrs. Smith's case would be able to tell *at a glance*:

1. That the condition had first been noted in her mid-twenties during pregnancy and had been noted again during a routine medical examination when she was 32 years old.
2. That there was a family history of hypertension and her father was diabetic.
3. That she had had recurrent urinary tract infections in the previous three years.
4. That she was overweight and there was a family history of obesity.
5. The provisional diagnosis.
6. What the targets are for systolic and diastolic blood pressures and weight.
7. The investigations which have already been done and those which may now be due.
8. The current treatment and the response of the blood pressure to it.
9. The pattern of weight reduction.
10. That she cannot be relied on to take her therapy or attend clinic regularly.
11. The fact that methyldopa produced side effects and had to be stopped.
12. The interval since the last review took place and whether it was of the recommended duration.

It would be interesting to know how often the above doctor would have elicited all these items of relevant information in the limited time available in a hospital or general practice consultation. Moreover, even if the doctor had been familiar with the patient he would have found this flow chart useful as an *aide memoire*, since doctors are usually less well-informed about their patients than they themselves believe.

REFERENCES

Abrams, M. E., *et al* (1968) A computer-based general practice and health centre information system, *Journal of the Royal College of General Practitioners*, **16**, 415–427.

Acheson, E. D., (1967) *Medical Record Linkage*, London: Oxford University Press.

Bjorn, J. C., & Cross, H. D., (1971) *The problem-orientated private practice of medicine*, Chicago: Modern Hospital Press.

British Medical Journal (1976) Leading article, **2**, 714.

Corbett, J. T. (1962) Keeping records in general practice, *Journal of the Royal College of General Practitioners*, **5**, 270–274.

Cormack, J. J. C., (1970) The medical record envelope – a case for reform. *Journal of the Royal College of General Practitioners*, **20**, 333–353.

Dawes, K. S., (1972) Survey of general practice records, *British Medical Journal*, **3**, 219–223.

Hodson, M., (1967) *Doctors and Patients*, London: Hodder and Stoughton.

Last, J. M., (1963) The iceberg – 'completing the clinical picture in general practice, *Lancet*, **ii**, 28–31.

Last, J. M., (1966) *International Medical Tribune of Great Britain*, **1**, No. 27 4.

Loudon, I. S. L., (1975) Record-keeping in general practice, *Update*, **10**, 259–266.

Nuffield Provincial Hospitals Trust, (1968) *Screening in Medical Care*, London: Oxford University Press.

Sheldon, M. G., (1974) An A4 size registration sheet for general practice, *Journal of the Royal College of General Practitioners*, **24**, 582–583.

Sheldon, M. G., (1976) Patient-filled questionnaires, *Update*, **13**, 651–660.

Tait, I., & Stevens, J., (1973) The problem-orientated medical record in general practice, *Journal of the Royal College of General Practitioners*, **23**, 311.

Tulloch, A. J., (1976) *The Design and Evaluation of a Modern Medical Record System*. M. D. thesis (unpublished), Aberdeen University.

Tulloch, A. J., (1976 a) Hospital Discharge Reports: Design and Content. *Update*, **13**, 517–520.

Weed, L. L., (1969) *Medical Records, Medical Education and Patient Care*, Cleveland: Press of Case Western Reserve University.

5

Educational aspects of the problem orientated medical record

GEOFFREY LLOYD[1] and NEIL McINTYRE[2]

Research Fellow, King's Fund Record Project, Academic Department of Medicine, Royal Free Hospital, London (now Medical Specialist, Ahmadi Hospital, Kuwait)
Reader, Academic Department of Medicine, Royal Free Hospital, Pond Street, London; Clinical Sub-Dean, Royal Free Hospital School of Medicine.

INTRODUCTION

First-hand knowledge is the ultimate basis for educational life. To a large extent book learning conveys secondhand information and as such can never rise to the importance of immediate practice. What the learned world tends to offer is one secondhand scrap of information illustrating ideas derived from another secondhand scrap of information. The secondhandedness of the learned world is the secret of its mediocrity. It is tame because it has never been scared by facts.

Alfred North Whitehead (1962)

The writing of clinical notes should be an important element in the training of medical students. Doctors' notes about patients are essential for the day to day practice of medicine and it would seem sensible that they should learn to write them when they are at medical school.

Students recognise the importance of keeping good records. In a survey of our own students more than 90 per cent considered full and accurate recording of clinical data to be an important characteristic of a good physician (Hughes, Lloyd and McIntyre, 1978). Unfortunately fewer (56 per cent) thought it an important characteristic of the good medical student and final year students valued it least.

In conventional student notes the sections on the history and physical examination are often well documented. There are two reasons for this. Firstly, their importance is stressed by teachers. Students know they must write them (even though their teachers may not bother to read them!). Secondly, both sections have a standard format with which both teachers and students are familiar.

But the rest of the record tends to be poorly documented. Students rarely record the results of special investigations and like their teachers they place little emphasis on management plans and progress notes – two important aspects of patient care. These sections of the notes have no agreed structure to guide the efforts of students in preparing them. It is hardly surprising that they are written badly, by doctors as well as by students.

We suspect that teachers neglect students' records because their own are so poor. The general standard of medical records is deplorable and few teachers are able to give sound advice to students about writing them. For this reason the problem orientated medical record (POMR) has proved a boon. It provides guidelines on writing clinical notes and deals not only with data collection (history taking, physical examination and results of laboratory investigations) but also with problem formulation, with planning of patient care and with follow-up.

POMR has been well received. In 1972, 82 American medical schools (out of 101) and 9 Canadian Schools (out of 16) were teaching the use of POMR (Adamson, 1974). It is used in several British medical schools (Metcalfe et al, 1977) and in schools in Australia, New Zealand, South Africa, Scandinavia and Israel. There are sections on POMR in standard textbooks of medicine (Goldfinger and Dineen, 1977; Johns, 1976) and paediatrics (McKay, 1975) and its use is advocated in a number of books which aim to introduce students to the principles of clinical methods (Enelow and Swisher, 1972; Morgan and Engel, 1969; Prior and Silberstein, 1973; Walker, Hall and Hurst, 1976). Weed did not publicise POMR until 1968 (Weed 1968, Weed 1969) and its rapid acceptance is a testimony to its attractiveness for many teachers.

The implications of POMR for medical education spread far beyond the improvement of medical records. We, like others (Walker, Hurst, Woody, 1973; Benbassat and Schiffmann, 1976; Neelon and Ellis, 1974), are enthusiastic about its use as an educational tool because it allows us to employ a powerful and effective teaching method.

We can ask a student to clerk a patient and to write up his own problem orientated record of his findings and plans. We can then take his notes and sit down with him to assess his performance, to comment on it and to help him to correct any deficiencies which we may find. Audit of the student's problem orientated medical record in this way is a powerful teaching method because it reflects the true goals of most clinical teachers. It is effective because it satisfies a number of important educational principles.

We would now like to discuss these goals and educational principles and illustrate how they can be promoted and satisfied by use of the problem orientated medical record.

GOALS, OBJECTIVES AND EDUCATIONAL PRINCIPLES

Goals and objectives

Medical schools are trying to produce 'good doctors' who can care for patients and who are ready for post-graduate specialist training. It is difficult to know whether they succeed because schools do not usually define what they mean by the term 'good doctor' nor do they specify the level of performance expected from students at the time of graduation. Some schools set goals for their students and usually they resemble the goals in Table 5.1 which were prepared by clinical teachers at the Royal Free Hospital School of Medicine.

These goals emphasise the skills of information collection and problem solving and stress the *application* of knowledge in the care of patients. They encourage students to admit ignorance but suggest that as independent learners they could minimise the effect of deficiencies by seeking help from appropriate sources and by continuing to learn during their years of active practice. The goals stress the importance of attitudes – towards patients, relatives and professional colleagues. There is little emphasis on the mere acquisition of facts.

Students should be given a copy of school goals and of any related departmental subgoals. We cannot expect them to master our goals unless they know what they are and what they must do in order to demonstrate mastery.

'Goals' are usually stated in rather vague terms – as broad statements of intent. For clarity we think it is also advisable to formulate more precise statements, called performance 'objectives', which describe what the student must *do* in order to demonstrate achievement of a goal (Mager, 1972; Mager, 1975). For one goal it may be necessary to write a number of objectives and it is important that they should match the intent of the goal (Mager, 1973). In these terms 'The student should be able to understand disorders of fluid and electrolyte metabolism' is clearly a goal. To match it the following objective might be written: 'Given the records of a postoperative patient the student should be able to write out a cumulative fluid-

Table 5.1 Broad goals agreed by teachers at the Royal Free Hospital School of Medicine.

At the end of the medical course students:-

1. Should be able to collect, record and communicate clinical information (i.e. data obtained from history, clinical examination and special investigations) in a thorough and reliable manner;
2. Should be able to use such information to solve and manage clinical problems;
3. Should have (without recourse to books) a core of knowledge and manipulative skills that will:-
    a. Facilitate their collection of clinical information,
    b. Enable them to handle acute, life threatening emergencies promptly and effectively,
    c. Allow them to deal efficiently with common clinical conditions,
    d. Give them an understanding of normal biological processes and how these are disturbed in disease states;
4. Should understand the potential influence of environmental and psychological factors on a patient's illness;
5. Should be familiar with the resources and facilities available through health and social services and be able to use them effectively for the benefit of their patients;
6. Should recognise the limitations of their own knowledge and abilities, admitting areas of ignorance and seeking help when necessary;
7. Should be familiar with scientific method and be able to apply scientific principles to the evaluation of published work;
8. Should be independent learners with attitudes to self evaluation and self education that will promote continuing improvement and adaptation to changes in medical practice, whether these result from the changing needs of the community or to advances in medical science;
9. Should be able to care for patients and their families – they should be able to reassure them, to allay their anxieties and to discuss illnesses and their treatment, prognosis and potential complications in terms which the patient and the family can understand (should be able to establish good relationships with patients and to communicate easily with them by the end of the first clinical year);
10. Should be able to establish good working relationships with their medical colleagues and members of allied health professions.

balance chart and to list the intravenous fluids and additives which would be appropriate therapy for the ensuing 24-hour period'. A little wordy, perhaps, but the intention is quite clear and the student is more likely to achieve this important objective (and so part of the goal) if it is spelled out for him in this fashion. Later we will present examples of performance objectives directly related to the use of POMR.

When goals and objectives are spelled out clearly students may be able to master them by their own efforts. But some can only be achieved effectively with intervention on the part of the teacher and this is true for several of the goals in Table 5.1.

Educational principles and methods

How should the teacher intervene in order to help the student? Our traditional methods of doing so leave much to be desired (Robson, 1973). There has been an overemphasis on facts and on their transmission by the lecture and by similar didactic techniques: only limited use is made of methods which help students to learn for themselves. We tend to rely on 'terminal' examinations and neglect continuing student assessment. Students feel obliged to hide their ignorance rather than to reveal it. All of these factors interfere with remedial teaching because they make it difficult for us to spot the need for it until it is too late. Even when the need is recognised it is difficult to help individual students because our methods make few allowances for varying interests, aptitudes and rates of learning.

We can help students in many ways. We can talk *to* them, talk *with* them or have them talk *together*. We can show them how to do things, supervise their own performance or provide opportunities for them to practise (Guilbert, 1976). But whatever we do, certain principles govern whether our teaching is effective, and these have been spelled out by Miller and his colleagues (Miller *et al*, 1961).

1. Learning is personal and can be done only be the student. It is activity on the part of the student which matters most, not activity on the part of the teacher. The teacher's job is to *promote* learning by increasing the students' motivation and by planning and coordinating the activities which will help them to achieve their educational goals and objectives. Currently we pay little attention to motivation of students as a key factor in helping them to learn.

2. Goals and objectives should be realistic. Students must be able to achieve them. If they continually fall short of their targets they tend to be frustrated and may be discouraged from further effort (Mager, 1968). They get pleasure from success which helps them to trust and respect their own abilities and to feel accepted by their teachers. When they are successful it is easier for them to admit their shortcomings and to accept constructive criticism.

3. Feedback is essential. This principle is particularly important. 'If he is not told whether he succeeds and has no means to judge for himself there is little point in making further efforts. Until the learner has established standards by which to assess his own performance he needs detailed and prompt criticism to redirect his learning.' (Beard, 1970).

Students often complain that feedback is inadequate; in our survey (Hughes *et al*, 1978) more than 80 per cent of our students said they were given little information on their progress. Feedback tends to be fragmentary and restricted to isolated points picked up when a student presents a patient or topic in front of a teacher. It may come too late for appropriate remedial action. Feedback must be prompt. . . . 'Progress in realising learning objectives must be constantly monitored, and the results *immediately* fed back to him in a form that is meaningful to both short term and long term action. The only really effective way of fulfilling this need is by means of regular and detailed counselling and guidance.' (Davies, 1971).

4. Teaching and learning should be based on good interpersonal relationships. Miller *et al* (1961) pointed out that students may learn from 'boors and martinets but most students withdraw from an environment which arouses in them strong emotions, anger, fear or frustration, and their learning suffers'. It is possible to improve relationships with our students if we are able to identify our deficiencies (Mager, 1968). We should encourage students to be open and critical and should permit confrontation. Learning should be seen as a cooperative and collaborative exercise in which imperfection is tolerated and mistakes viewed as opportunities for correction. We should make students feel accepted and respected and should encourage them to evaluate themselves. It is not easy to do this when dealing with a group of students and it is helpful if students and teachers can meet on a one-to-one basis.

5. Teaching should be relevant. It should help to fit students for tasks which lie ahead and in the case of medical students it must help them, directly or indirectly, to learn to care for patients. Students must see the connection between what is taught and what they must eventually be able to do; otherwise their motivation to learn will be limited, their attention will stray and they will learn little.

Not only must information be relevant it must also be acquired by students in a relevant context. Facts learned by reading or in lectures or tutorials tend to be quickly forgotten. They are much better remembered if they are applied in practice and if they are reinforced by frequent usage. Therefore the information should be used in solving clinical problems so that learning occurs in the context of clinical practice.

We have discussed goals and objectives, and the principles of learning at some length. A good teaching method should help us to promote our goals and help our students to master their objectives; it should also observe the educational principles spelled out above. On this basis audit of the students' problem orientated records seems to us to be an admirable method of promoting learning. As we shall see in the next section it helps to promote virtually all the goals presented in Table 5.1. Its objectives are realistic. It calls for the student's own efforts in simulating the care of patients; thus it is personal and highly relevant. It involves teacher and student in one-to-one sessions (which improve interpersonal relationships); rapid feedback is given and it allows us to teach at a level appropriate to the individual student. The theoretical advantages of such a strategy are obvious. More importantly we have found that it works in practice, although it does require that students and teachers assume different roles from those usually adopted.

THE ROLE OF THE STUDENT

If students are to help to make this method a success they must realise why audit of their notes is such an important part of their clinical training. Learning to care for patients properly is a complex business. It is not enough to be able to handle parts of the process, such as history taking, physical examination or diagnosis. The student must practise the whole process. He can do this by simulating the total care of the patients whom he clerks during his undergraduate training. Initially, he will make mistakes, but if his notes record his intended management as well as his findings we can review this; we can point out his errors, praise his successes, and give useful feedback in order to improve his subsequent performance.

Audit is useful in another way. Ignorance is one of the least important causes of error in clinical medicine; most mistakes stem from poor organisation, failure of communication, laziness or carelessness (Gruver and Freis, 1959; Pyke, 1976). These are defects of behaviour not of knowledge. The student's notes can help us to assess and therefore to promote good behaviour. We can check his thoroughness, reliability, analytical sense and efficiency. These matter more· than the number of facts he can remember.

What then must the student do? He must clearly give a high priority to clerking his patients. He must collect information about them thoroughly and reliably and should use this information to simulate management. He must decide what problems require activity or attention, should plan for them and follow them up until they are resolved or until he loses contact with the patient. He must decide what he would tell the patient and what reply to give to the patient's queries. In short he must act like a doctor. We can check the student's performance if he writes up his findings, his conclusions and his plans in a problem orientated format. For this purpose a good record is essential. It tells us what the student 'did' – not what he knew and this allows us to assess his 'core of behaviour'.

To clarify what is expected of students we have written some performance objectives to match the goals of Table 5.1. Two of these relate directly to the use of POMR and to audit of the student's performance. They are clearly important and we believe that it is worth spelling them out in detail.

A. *The student will demonstrate that he collects information thoroughly* by recording for all his in-patients those details of history, physical examination and laboratory investigation which are routinely collected on the firm to which he is attached.

The history should include a statement of the presenting complaint, the history of the present illness, the results of a systematic enquiry and past, family, psychosocial and drug histories. The student should, when necessary, incorporate information obtained from sources other than the patient, such as family or earlier medical records.

The physical examination should describe all items stated in the data base for each firm. It should include:- general description of the patient, skin examination, examination of cardiovascular system, respiratory system, abdomen, central and peripheral nervous systems, the musculoskeletal system and psychiatric examination.

The record of laboratory investigations should note all routine requests and the results of these as they return.

Assessment will be made throughout the post by inspection of a random selection of his clinical notes on current in-patients. Acceptable performance is the *complete* collection of the clinical information expected routinely by the teachers responsible for the individual firms.

B. *The student will demonstrate his ability to interpret and utilise clinical information.* In his clinical notes on each in-patient he should:

1. formulate from his data base a list of significant problems which require activity and attention;

2. construct for each of these active problems a plan of action. This should include the collection of further information to help diagnosis and/or monitoring of patients. He should describe the treatment he recommends, write the names of the drugs in block capitals and give the dosage and route of administration (as in a prescription). He should record how he would involve health care workers or social services. He should describe the advice he would give to the patient and record the patient's fears about his illness and its consequences;

3. record the progress of each problem, noting changes in symptoms and physical signs and the results of investigations as they return. If tests which he recommended were not carried out, he should indicate why these were not done (having consulted the medical staff). He should record his assessment of the status of problems as

new information returns. He should write plans for further investigations or changes of treatment. He should monitor his patient for potential complications of therapy, including predictable hazards of usage, side effects and drug interactions. When monitoring intravenous fluid therapy, a cumulative chart of fluid and electrolyte balance should be recorded.

The student's performance will be acceptable if his reasoning is clear in the notes and in discussion with his teachers, and if he can defend his statements and decisions on the basis of common sense, established practice or by reference to authoritative sources such as recent texts, journals, drug information leaflets, Prescribers Journals, the National Formulary or pharmacopoeias.

The student's clinical performance will be displayed in the four main sections of POMR – the data base, problem list, plans and progress notes. Each describes a different aspect of patient care and calls for different efforts on the part of the student. When writing his problem orientated notes the student should imagine himself as the doctor in charge of the patient. He should record his own findings, formulate his own problem list, and write his own plans and progress notes. When he can tackle all of these tasks he will be well on his way to providing patients with care of a high quality.

The data base
Students should aim to collect a complete data base on each of their in-patients. They can do this only if they know what information they must collect routinely on any given clinical attachment i.e. what constitutes a 'complete' data base. This should be spelled out for them. They should know why each piece of information is collected and the significance of a positive response. They must realise that the amount of information collected will depend on the type of patient seen by a doctor, on his work load and on the resources available to him. They will then understand why the 'defined data base' is not the same on all posts and will be able to decide on their own data base when, eventually, they need to do so (See Ch. 2).

With our traditional approach to data collection students are rarely clear about the amount of information which they *must* collect and 'standards' vary accordingly. They have a rough idea about the content of a history and physical examination but often leave out important items without reflecting on the possible consequences.

Students themselves like to be told what information they should collect routinely particularly when they are beginning clinical studies. It enables them to take histories and to do physical examinations at a time when they might otherwise be handicapped by uncertainty. When they collect and record a 'complete' data base students get practice in asking many different questions and in clarifying the answers; they practise the physical examination of the different body systems and regularly review the results of routine investigations. They learn how to frame questions so that they are understood by patients and discover the range of patient responses. They learn which questions give the greatest yield. Gradually, they gain confidence in their ability not only to record the presenting complaint but also to pick up problems which have previously been unidentified.

Traditionally students have ignored the review of investigations even if they are ordered routinely on a particular post. This neglect is serious. Routine tests frequently unearth asymptomatic problems which require action or which deserve recognition even if no action is called for. It is obviously important that students should become thoroughly familiar with the purpose of these tests and with their consequences. If the tests are done routinely then the students should handle the results routinely. It is one of the strengths of the problem orientated approach that the history, physical examination and special investigations are *all* recorded as part of the 'defined data base'.

Students should collect a data base as soon as possible after the patient's admission to hospital. They will then be involved in the acute situation and can follow the patient throughout his hospital stay. But sometimes students do not contact the patient for several days. Curiously, when they write the history of the present illness they still tend to close it at the moment of admission and ignore (in the notes) significant events which have occurred in hospital. We believe that this is an artificial approach which should be discouraged. Instead, students should continue the story up to the time at which they first see the patient (as a houseman does when he writes up a patient transferred from another hospital); they should include the results of investigations which have returned and should record treatment already given. They can then make their own plans for further care – not artificial ones which might have been appropriate (with hindsight) several days before.

The problem list
Traditionally, teachers have stressed the importance of 'diagnosing' the main complaints. Students have been asked to commit themselves to 'one answer' even if it could be little more than an educated guess. In trying to elucidate the cause of the major complaint they have often ignored other clinical features. But these may have needed treatment

in their own right or may have had powerful interactions with the main complaints.

We believe that such emphasis on a single diagnosis is misguided. Students should learn to identify all abnormalities in the data base and to analyse them to find problems deserving attention. Having done so, they should construct a problem list. Abnormalities belonging together should be grouped under a single heading while the remainder should be considered as separate problems to be listed and dealt with individually. During the construction of a problem list the students should avoid 'guesses' and 'hypotheses'. Problems should be formulated as statements of fact which are substantiated by the available information. Students should list *all* problems. They need to see how problems interrelate and how one problem affects the management of others.

Problem formulation is a difficult but instructive process. Arguably it is the most important task of the doctor, for if problems are not correctly identified it is virtually impossible to make appropriate plans for helping the patient (an argument also put forward by those who advocate 'diagnosis' rather than problem formulation).

Some teachers disparage the construction of a problem list. They argue that it is artificial to review the patient's record and to make a problem list because it is not how doctors normally work. They claim, with reason, that diagnostic hypotheses are generated early in the taking of a history, and that these hypotheses influence what information is collected during the interview (Elstein *et al*, 1972).

Such arguments do not hold for students early in their period of training. Without experience they cannot formulate and act on hypotheses while they are listening to the patient's story. For students, it is necessary to review patients' records if they are to learn how to generate hypotheses, to identify common patterns of symptoms and signs, and to discriminate between important pieces of information ('signals') and those which are unimportant ('noise').

But even for doctors review of the record is important. Both our ability to make judgements and our span of immediate memory are very restricted; they impose severe limitations on the amount of information that we are able to receive, process and remember (Miller, 1956). This explains why we tend to concentrate on certain areas of the patient's clinical picture and why, if we rely on our memories, we must ignore others. But many patients have complicated illnesses. They may have lots of symptoms and signs and a plethora of abnormal laboratory results. They may suffer from many different conditions all of which require our attention. If we are to consider each problem on its merits then we must supplement our memories and to do this we need a written record. Record review is essential, but at present it is a practice which is widely neglected. If we are to promote such an approach to patient care then we should emphasise its importance during undergraduate training. We can do it by encouraging students to review their notes, to formulate problems and to produce a problem list.

Plans

After formulating a problem list, students must decide what action they will take. They must make *plans*. Problem orientated plans have a substructure covering four main areas of clinical activity. First, if a problem is stated at a lower level than a precise diagnosis, for example, dyspnoea, splenomegaly or hypokalaemia, students must generate higher level hypotheses, for example, left heart failure, cirrhosis of the

```
STEATORREOEA

    Dx    ? COELIAC DISEASE - JEJUNAL BIOPSY

          ? PANCREATIC DISEASE - PANCREATIC SCAN

                              - LUNDH TEST ON PANCREATIC JUICE

          ? BACTERIAL CONTAMINATION - Ba meal, follow through

                                    - 14 C GLYCOCHOLATE BREATH TEST

                                    - SERUM B 12



    Mx    3 DAY FAECAL FAT

          DAILY STOOL WEIGHT

    Ex    Investigations to check cause of diarrhoea.  Optimistic

          that treatable cause will be found.
```

Fig. 5.1 An initial plan.

liver or Conn's syndrome respectively, and suggest *further information* to support or refute them. Each diagnostic hypothesis should be clearly linked to the special investigations, or other bits of information, which would support or refute it, as in Fig. 5.1. This procedure should not be neglected. We often find that students (and doctors!) do not understand why tests are done on their patients. They do not appreciate the diagnostic value of the tests and may be unaware of the way in which a particular problem should be investigated. Regular practice at linking tests and hypotheses helps to improve their diagnostic ability.

Secondly, students must *monitor* their patients' progress. They must decide what observations or tests they will make and should indicate how often they will call for them. During audit they might be asked to justify the cost or to defend their choice on other grounds. At present monitoring is sadly neglected in undergraduate and post-graduate education.

The third section of problem orientated plans covers *therapy*. In the second objective we have stated clearly how we expect students to lay out their therapeutic plans.

The fourth section relates to *patient education*. Here the student should record what he would tell the patient about the problem; he should record relevant comments made by the patient e.g. whether the patient thinks he has cancer or whether the patient's attitude to a problem is inappropriate. This section is particularly important as it should help to ensure that the student will communicate with the patient, and will record this communication for his own benefit and for that of others. This area is virtually ignored in conventional clinical training and it is not surprising that patients complain about our failure to communicate with them.

Students should construct their own plans and not copy those of the houseman or registrar. The students' initial plans should deal with problems as they present at the time of writing not as they may have presented on admission. If an ECG and enzyme determination have already confirmed a myocardial infarction then a student should plan solely for its management and not 'pretend' to be investigating chest pain. He should decide what complications to look out for and indicate how he would monitor the patient for them. He should describe necessary treatment and record how he would explain the significance of the infarction to the patient. In this way the student maintains contact with reality. When his actions differ from those of the houseman, registrar or consultant he should try to discover why.

Students should spend time on their initial plans – reading or seeking advice when they are uncertain about the best course of action. The importance of planning cannot be overemphasised as it makes the student use the information at his disposal.

Progress notes

After plans have been constructed, students must be encouraged to follow up their patients and to write progress notes about them. The process of clinical care is not finished when a diagnosis is made or when treatment has been started. Students should be able to assess the results of therapy and to decide whether further investigations are needed or whether treatment should be changed. They should plan the patient's return home, 'recruit' the help of the social services and decide on the frequency of follow-up. These are important aspects of medical care and the students' training should take account of them. The basic format of problem orientated progress notes provides guidelines for the students about the way in which in-patients should be followed up.

Students cannot restrict their learning to the clerking of their patients in the way outlined above. They must do many other things during their clinical under-graduate training. They could not become skilled in the interpretation of physical signs only by examining their own patients. Their experience needs to be supplemented and they must seek and examine patients with abnormal physical signs. They must read about many common conditions as it is unlikely that each student will be allocated patients who, collectively, have all the common and important conditions with which he should become familiar during his under-graduate training. Students must learn about X-rays, about ECGs, and about aspects of medicine such as epidemiology, and about some important principles of pathology which appear to be divorced from the immediate problems of clinical care. To teach these different aspects we need to use a variety of educational techniques. All of them may be important but we believe that audit of the student's management of patients should be given the highest priority.

THE ROLE OF THE TEACHER

In the previous section we described the performance required from students. The teacher has two tasks. Firstly, he must check that students' work is acceptable and that it matches the criteria laid out in the objectives. Secondly, he must help the student to correct any deficiencies that are found.

When students clerk their patients using the POMR, we are able to evaluate their overall clinical performance. We can check the thoroughness with which they collect clinical information (if the criteria for complete collection have been defined) and we can check the reliability of their findings. Their analytical sense will be displayed by the way in which they construct problem lists, plans and progress notes.

An example of a student's problem list is presented in Fig. 5.2a. This student had omitted several important items from his problem list – penicillin sensitivity, long-term steroid therapy, bilateral cataracts, a systolic murmur, high blood glucose and high blood urea. He had noted all of them in his data base but had not formulated them as problems and so had made no plans for them. These omissions were pointed out. He dealt with them and learned how to monitor and manage patients on long-term steroids, discovered that the high blood urea was due to fluid depletion and that the systolic murmur was caused by mitral incompetence. He attributed the high blood glucose to the steroid therapy and dealt with the cataracts by suggesting referral to an opthalmologist.

Initially he wrote plans only for the asthma (Fig. 5.2b). There were

	Active Problems	Inactive Problems
1	Asthma	
2		Removal of Nasal Polyps 1963 and 1970
3		Myocardial Infarct - Jan 1977
4		*Allergy to Penicillin*
5	*Long term steroid therapy*	
6	*Bilateral cataracts*	
7	*Systolic murmur*	
8	*High blood glucose*	
9	*High blood urea*	

Fig. 5.2a. A problem list prepared by a student early in his first clinical year. The first three problems in normal type were listed as problems by the student. Those in italics were added during audit from information present in the data base which he collected.

ASTHMA

Dx	2° to emotional upset
	? L.V.F.
	? chest infection - sputum culture + microscopy,
	- Gram stain.
Mx	Peak flow twice daily
	28% O_2
	Physiotherapy
	Fluid chart
Rx	Maintain present therapy
	Amoxycillin 250 mg t.d.s.

Fig. 5.2b The student's initial plans relating to the problem list presented above.

many faults in these plans which reflected his limited understanding of the diagnosis and management of asthmatic attacks. He did not indicate how he would decide whether the patient was in left ventricular failure. He mixed up treatment and the collection of information for monitoring. His description of therapy was poor; there was no entry for patient education. With feedback on these faults his subsequent performance improved markedly.

By reviewing students' notes, we can check many other aspects of the students' ability. We can evaluate their understanding of the effect of environmental and psychological factors on a patient's illness (*See* Goal 4 - Table 5.1), their familiarity with and ability to use the resources of the Health and Social Services (Goal 5), and through their comments on 'patient education' their understanding of the interaction between doctor and patient (Goal 9). We can assess the students' critical faculties (Goal 7) from the way in which they apply to patient care information gleaned from textbooks and other sources. We can assess their development as independent learners (Goal 8) and the extent to which they appreciate the limitations of their own knowledge (Goal 6). Goals 1 and 2 are covered more directly by the problem orientated approach. Thus audit of the POMR allows us to evaluate and so to promote most of our school goals.

Audit of the students' notes is best done on a one-to-one basis as students dislike criticism in front of other students. Some authors believe that auditor's comments should be written out and that students should reply in writing (Voytovich, 1973). We prefer to sit down with an individual student in order to review one of his records. We can then work at the level of his ability; he may require the correction of simple faults or he may be capable of discussing detailed and complicated aspects of management. This individualised approach improves student/teacher relationships, furthers the 'apprenticeship' aspect of clinical training and allows misunderstandings to be corrected quickly and easily.

The set of notes used for audit should as far as possible be chosen at random. If the student does not know which patient's notes will be looked at, we can assume that his behaviour and standard of performance will be similar in his handling of other patients.

The success of audit will depend on the way in which it is conducted. Students should view audit as an educational process designed to improve performance and not as something punitive. Rules should be agreed beforehand so that the teachers' judgements are seen to be consistent and to be rational and fair. There will then be less chance of disagreement, criticisms will appear less threatening and it is more likely that they will be accepted as constructive.

Initially we use audit sessions to try to improve the student's use of the problem orientated record; it is the best method of teaching POMR. Some critics object to our emphasis on the structure of the record and argue that we should concentrate on its content. But if the structure is poor it may be difficult to evaluate the content. As students learn to use POMR properly we find that the content of their notes tends to improve dramatically and we attribute this to the quality of the problem orientated structure as a guidance system.

Except for teaching on the record itself, we try not to instruct students or to supply them with information. Instead we encourage students to seek information themselves and help them to learn how to find it. We aim to make students into independent learners and try to promote habits which will support them when they have left our influence. Students must learn that the ability to handle and solve clinical problems is a skill which must be developed by practice and that it does not come automatically with an increase in factual knowledge. We discourage students from rote learning as the half-life of information picked up in this way is short (Buzan, 1974). We encourage them to consult reference sources frequently while they are writing up their notes. In this way they learn to use reference sources properly and we hope that they will eschew the use of books designed as 'crammers'; such books are rarely of value in handling real clinical problems.

Many good clinicians are poor teachers when they use conventional teaching methods. They may lecture badly and be poor instructors at the bedside. But they may excel during audit when their job is not to transmit information but to comment on the student's own performance. Then clinical skills and experience come to the fore.

Audit can be used by teachers of many different disciplines. Clinical pathologists and radiologists can check the student's handling of the information which they provide. They can ensure that students understand why certain bits of information are collected routinely and that they know the likely causes of abnormalities and how they should be followed up. They can help students to use the laboratory well.

The POMR is a particularly powerful tool for the clinical pharmacologist, who can study the way in which students simulate the prescription of drugs. In our objectives we ask that a student 'should describe the treatment he recommends. He should write the names of drugs in block capitals and give dosage and route of administration (as in a prescription). He should monitor for potential complications of therapy, including predictable hazards of usage, side-effect and drug interactions'. The advantages of this approach seem obvious. It allows the clinical pharmacologist (and his clinical colleagues) to promote therapeutic skills and ensures that the student concentrates his efforts on common forms of therapy.

Emphasis on audit of the students' records as a method of teaching involves a major change in educational approach. Traditionally we have evaluated the students' recall of factual information; we have not checked whether they can apply knowledge in practice or whether they *do* things which they know should be done. We can do this with audit. If teachers are able to adopt this new approach to clinical education we think it will have profound effects on students' performance and on their subsequent performance as doctors. For like Ruskin (quoted in Rowntree, 1974), we believe that 'education does not mean teaching people to know what they do not know. It means teaching them to behave as they do not behave'.

IMPLEMENTATION

It is not an easy matter to implement the educational method outlined in the preceding sections. Problems are many and difficult. We have audited students' POMR for several years and during the last year, with other teachers at the Royal Free Hospital School of Medicine, we have used audit in association with a new clinical curriculum which came into force in October, 1976. Before that time we conducted a trial of audit as a form of in-course assessment. It was evaluated, using an illuminative approach to evaluation (Parlett and Hamilton, 1975) by two educationalists from the University of Surrey. In their report (Dearden and Laurillard, 1976) they concluded that 'Its teaching value and potential as a method for in-course assessment has shone through the inevitable management difficulties'. But they stressed that problems of organisation and communication occurred throughout the trial and could have overwhelmed it. That they did not was atrributed to frequent staff-student meetings which allowed grievances to be aired and examined. Dearden and Laurillard wrote that although there were many problems which required serious consideration they believed that they could be solved.

Before the new clinical curriculum was introduced at the Royal Free the curriculum committee agreed that we should evaluate its effect and its progress. This evaluation is being carried out jointly by Janet Gale, an educational psychologist from the British Life Assurance Trust (BLAT) Centre for Health and Medical Education, and Elizabeth Wyn Pugh, a gynaecologist, also from the BLAT Centre, who is a graduate of the Royal Free Hospital School of Medicine and who has worked with our clinical teachers on the specification of our goals and objectives. Their reports cover all aspects of the new curriculum and include many comments about the use of POMR and of audit.

Students beginning clinical studies in October 1976 were taught how to use the POMR during an Introductory Course (which also covered other topics) and were asked to employ it subsequently on all attachments which involved the clerking of patients. Their performance has been monitored by audit from the beginning.

Unfortunately the Introductory Course did not give students an adequate grounding in the principles of POMR (teaching on POMR was limited to two lessons involving the whole class of approximately 100 students). Furthermore, our new curriculum was implemented hastily (for several reasons) and no programme was set up to ensure that all first year teachers were fully informed about the new curriculum. Few of them were familiar with POMR or with the advice which students had been given during the Introductory Course. This led to many difficulties. During the first six months of the new curriculum students have been confused about writing POMR and have not always been able to get clarification from teachers on their own posts. Advice is available to them within the hospital but students are either reluctant to seek it or remain unaware of how to get this advice. Our evaluators have suggested that sources of advice about POMR must be made more available to students and this we plan to do. They have also suggested that greater emphasis should be placed on writing and using POMR in the Introductory Course. We hope to improve teaching on POMR in the Introductory Course and have prepared a short self-instructional booklet on the writing of problem lists, plans and progress notes (Lloyd and Anthony-Samy, 1977).

It is important that students should learn to use POMR in the early stages of their clinical training. Then they can easily master the problem orientated approach. But if they learn bad habits initially it may be difficult for them to adjust subsequently to the discipline involved in its correct use.

The attitudes of teachers to POMR are critical in determining the success of problem orientated audit. A small number of teachers are against POMR. Asked why, they give a variety of reasons. They may object to its complexity, artificiality or rigidity, or they may argue that it has the wrong philosophical basis. Some complain that it uses up too much paper or that the effort involved is unnecessarily great. Others claim that it takes students away from patients, that it leads to a fragmentation of problems, or that it leads to failure to identify priorities. Even teachers who accept POMR may feel that some of these objections are justified. We would argue that such attitudes to POMR stem from a misunderstanding of the principles of POMR and from exposure to poor examples of its use.

We need to convince such teachers that the use of POMR is beneficial. Our evaluators recommended that teachers should be given ample opportunities to learn about POMR, and that sources of advice about POMR should be made readily available to them. But it is not an easy matter to reach clinical teachers. They are usually very busy and are often reluctant to read about or to attend sessions on teaching, on their methods of practice or on medical records. This is an educational dilemma. Fortunately, many of our teachers have indicated that they would welcome some training in the use of the POMR.

Our evaluators have noted several commonly expressed worries about the problem orientated approach and about audit of the record. Some teachers are concerned that in our new curriculum students spend too much time collecting information and too little using it; that they devote too much time to writing notes and too little to their patients. Some criticise the use of a 'defined data base' which outlines for each clinical post the information which they are expected to collect routinely from patients. They argue that its predefined content leads to a stereotyped approach to data collection and that students collect a large number of answers without understanding their implications. This criticism is rather surprising. The description of the patient's presenting illness is no different from that found in traditional notes which also include systematic questioning, a past history and family, psychosocial and drug histories; traditional notes also contain a fairly standard physical examination. The problem orientated data base is only different because

1. its content has been made explicit,
2. some ward and laboratory tests are included as routine requirements along with a history and physical examination.

The size and content of each defined data base used in our new curriculum were decided by the consensus of senior teachers on each post. It was made clear that the data base could be shortened if teachers felt it was too long and after the first three months of the curriculum teachers were invited to review their data bases. Few changes were made.

Students consider the data bases invaluable for indicating what clinical information should be collected on each post. It is not true that they do not understand the implications of the questions which they ask. During the first year our students have been asked to read about the symptoms, physical signs and laboratory results with which they deal routinely in their data bases. At the end of each three months they have been given a set of non-cued, short answer questions which check whether they appreciate the likely significance of any abnormalities which they may find (Fig. 5.3). Their performance in these tests has been most encouraging.

Information about patients continues to accrue after the initial work up and will include the results of tests requested for diagnostic purposes or for monitoring. The problem orientated approach stresses the recording of these data which are important and highly relevant to patient care. We cannot accept that the student who collects them is moving away from the patient. Quite the contrary. Of course we agree that data must be used and not simply collected, but would argue that the *correct* application of the problem orientated approach guarantees appropriate use. It requires students to *use* information in order to formulate problems and to construct initial plans. When they

1/ A patient's haematology report gives the following results:

Hb 7 g/dl,   PCV 21.8, MCV 105 Fl, MCHC 32 g/dl.

a) How would you describe this haematological finding,

b,c) Give 2 causes.

a)

b)

c)

2/ A 56-year old man who has smoked 30 cigarettes per day for years presents with a persistent cough, recent haemoptysis and increasing breathlessness.   Give 3 likely causes.

a)

b)

c)

3/ A 50-year old Pakistani female presents with localised lymphadenopathy in the lower half of the left posterior triangle of the neck.   Give 3 likely causes.

a)

b)

c)

Fig. 5.3 Examples of end of post questions.

receive the results of tests they must incorporate these in their notes, along with changes in symptoms and physical signs; they do this in order to assess the patient's progress and to make further plans. The major emphasis of the problem orientated approach is on information *handling* not on information *collection*. That information collection is also stressed is not surprising. Unless the information is collected it cannot be used.

Audit has been of concern to many teachers. Initially their greatest worry was about the time required for audit but this criticism is heard less often after experience of the new curriculum. We recommend that an audit should not last longer than thirty minutes. On a firm of eight students four hours of teacher time are needed to audit each student once a week. As all the teachers can audit (including consultants, registrars, lecturers, etc.) we find that few teachers spend more than an hour a week on audit. This has proved an acceptable load and it is no longer a serious logistic problem except on one or two understaffed posts.

There is sometimes a bonus for the teacher in one-to-one audit. When he reviews the student's notes on one of his own patients he may uncover information of which he was unaware. This allows him to correct mistakes or to institute new forms of treatment and the patient may benefit accordingly.

Some teachers claim that audit reduces the time available for bedside teaching and we accept this as an undesirable consequence. But audit occupies only half an hour of the student's time and not more than an hour of a teacher's time each week. If something has to give in order to allow audit to take place, we suggest that time should be taken from teaching sessions in which the student plays a relatively passive role.

But while time is less of a problem, timetabling is still difficult. Arrangements have to be made for teachers and students to meet at a mutually convenient time and this has to be done week in, week out, throughout the course. Both teachers and students are subject to many other pressures and it is hardly surprising that neither group can be relied on to organise regular audits if arrangements are made on an ad hoc basis. It is particularly difficult for students to initiate audits as they tend to be shy of approaching members of staff.

Hospital life is such that audits often have to be cancelled at short notice and it may be difficult for students and teachers to make contact in order to fix a new time. These problems were clearly identified in our trial scheme early in 1976 (Dearden and Laurillard, 1976). For the new curriculum we arranged central facilities to help students and teachers in arranging audits. These did improve matters but they were not used to full advantage during the first six months. Only a minority of posts have organised audits successfully. On most posts, audits have proved difficult to arrange, have been difficult to keep because of other work, and have been difficult to rearrange. The goal of one audit a week has not yet been attained. But we are optimistic. Attitudes towards audit are improving and there is growing willingness on the part of students and staff to make sure that audits occur.

Both teachers and students have expressed uncertainty about the purpose of audits. In a document issued to all teachers on 'In-Course Assessment' (ICA) the clinical curriculum committee stressed that ICA (including audits) should be used primarily for feedback to students about their performance and only secondarily as a means of testing students in order to score them for eventual certification.

Students and staff rate the teaching element of audit highly and greatly appreciate the way in which it helps teachers to get to know their students. Our evaluators commented that 'Students have

CHECKLIST FOR AUDITORS

DATE
day   month   year
_____

Student _____
Patient _____
Auditor _____
Subject _____

COLLECTION OF INFORMATION

History of presenting illness   thorough ☐
                                                           reliable ☐
                                                           thorough ☐
                                                           reliable ☐
                                                           thorough ☐
                                                           reliable ☐

Laboratory investigations   *thorough* ☐

FORMULATION OF PROBLEMS

                                     Construction of problem list ☐
                                           analytically sound ☐

PLANS   *Structure and thoroughness* ☐
Diagnostic information   analytically sound ☐
Monitoring information   analytically sound ☐
Therapy   analytically sound ☐
Patient education   analytically sound ☐

PROGRESS NOTES

                                     Structure and thoroughness ☐
                                           analytically sound ☐

      Satisfactory performance   +
      Unsatisfactory performance   −

      In individual cases you may be unable to audit certain items;
      if so, please put N/A.

      If short of time, you may omit to audit the items in italics
      as these can be audited by others.

Fig. 5.4

enjoyed and benefited from audit more than most teachers may have imagined'.

But the 'assessment' component of audit causes concern and there is little enthusiasm for it. This stems from several factors. In our initial trial of audit we used an audit form in which the acceptability of the student's performance was scored as plus or minus (Fig. 5.4). Students were unhappy about the implications of the minus sign and so we changed to plus and zero. They then pointed out that this simple score allowed no indication of whether their performance was improving.

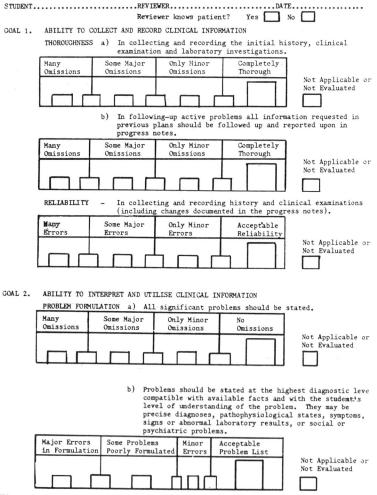

Fig. 5.5a

Consequently for our new curriculum we designed a new form with a seven point scale (Fig. 5.5a and 5.5b). Trials with a small number of auditors seemed satisfactory; the form appeared self-explanatory and we introduced it without explaining its use to new auditors. This failure of communication was costly. Auditors state that they do not understand the form and tend to miss out sections or to allot ticks rather uncertainly. Individual auditors have developed their own system of use and as a result their scoring has been highly variable. This variability has been confirmed by asking a number of auditors to rate the same record.

Some teachers make allowance for students' inexperience. If they think the students have tried hard they may give high ratings which are not justified by the students' actual performance. As the student gains more experience his performance improves but the auditor's scores remain the same because his expectation of student performance has also risen. While this approach is intended as a kindness to the student, it vitiates the purpose of the form.

PLANS FOR ACTIVE PROBLEMS AND PLANS IN PROGRESS NOTES

DIAGNOSIS : Indicates appropriate diagnostic hypotheses.

| Many Errors and Omissions | Some Major Errors Or Omissions | Only Minor Errors Or Omissions | Appropriate Hypotheses | Not Applicable Not Evaluated |

FURTHER INFORMATION COLLECTION : Suggests appropriate tests and further information required to establish diagnosis and/or to monitor the progress of the problem.

| Many Errors and Omissions | Some Major Errors Or Omissions | Only Minor Errors Or Omissions | Appropriate Requests | Not Applicable Not Evaluated |

THERAPY : Describes all forms of therapy appropriate and records drugs (using proper names written in block capitals and stating dose and route of administration.

| Seriously Inappropriate Therapy | Some Major Errors or Omissions | Only Minor Errors or Omissions | Appropriate Therapy | Not Applicable or Not Evaluated |

PATIENT EDUCATION : Describe where appropriate, the advice he would give the patient and records patients fears about his illness.

| Omitted or Seriously Inappropriate | Some Errors or Omissions | Minor Omissions | Present and Appropriate | Not Applicable or Not Evaluated |

Fig. 5.5b

Because of these several difficulties we have been unable to use the results of audits to tell students about their progress over a period of manŷ months. Of course they do get feedback during each audit, and most auditors discuss with the students the score given for each section of the form, but we believe that students would like to see 'objective' evidence of their improvement. It has also been difficult to use the scores of audits to assess whether the problem orientated approach helps students to learn clinical management, although many of our auditors are convinced of its value. This is a pity. Nelson and his colleagues (1976) used audit of similar kind and from the scores were able to demonstrate changes in student performance. If it can be made to work it is clearly a powerful educational tool if only for this reason.

There is a final problem with the form currently in use. We wish the student to appreciate priorities in patient care but this is not taken into account by the present form. A patient may have two serious problems and several problems of less importance. The student may perform admirably on the serious problems but do badly on the others. If the auditors stick strictly to current rules students score poorly because of mistakes or omissions in handling the lesser problems. Such an end

a) GUIDELINES FOR AUDITORS
      The following are guidelines that we have found useful in avoiding unnecessary pitfalls. Since we do not have any particular expertise to call upon, we have had to rely on a trial and error method. These then are the product of our collective but limited experience and must in no way be construed as rules.

1. Audit one student at a time. If a group audit is used for teaching purposes, it is unwise to assess a particular student in that group.
2. If there is more than one set of notes offered by the student then select the notes yourself rather than have the student make the choice.
3. Try as far as possible to use notes of patients that are currently in the ward.
4. Don't exceed 45 minutes for any one audit session. The average duration should be between 20 and 30 minutes.
5. When a deficiency in performance is noted, institute corrective action yourself or tell the student how to correct the deficiency.
6. Try to avoid the "mini-lecture" approach especially if the subject matter is adequately covered in a recommended text.
7. Students should be encouraged to go to a specialist auditor when an obvious biochemical, haematological or psychiatric abnormality exists in their patient.
8. Auditors should negotiate scores with the student and must always be prepared to answer questions.

b) DEFINITIONS OF THE TERMS USED IN THE AUDIT FORMS

1. Thoroughness:
      a) Complete collection of the routine data agreed for that firm and specified in the objectives.
      b) Complete collection of information related to the presenting complaint(s) as outlined in the checklists.
      c) A plan for each active problem (however brief).
      d) Follow-up of all intentions recorded in the plans.

2. Reliability:
      Accurate account of history and accurate detection of physical signs.

3. Analytical Sense:
      The ability to defend statements in the record on the basis of common sense, accepted medical practice or reference to a recent text or journal.

Fig. 5.6

result is clearly inappropriate and our form needs amendment to clear up this discrepancy. In discussion with the student the auditor should concentrate on the major problems and also on the most serious defects in the student's performance. The importance of priorities must always be stressed.

Our evaluators have recommended that we change our audit forms. They have also stressed that the 'rules of audit' must be clear in the minds of teachers and students as it is uncertainty about these rules which has led to many of our problems. We have prepared guidelines and definitions for the auditors (Fig. 5.6). It is particularly important that we should clarify how audit contributes to the overall grades which the students are given for ICA. Students recognise the educational value of audit but such appreciation develops only as a result of regular audit. If students believed that audits were not taken into account for overall ICA grades some might not bother to turn up for audit. This has indeed been our experience with a handful of students. To counter this we have awarded an 'unacceptable' grade for particularly poor attendance and this has been communicated to the students concerned. This procedure has proved effective in keeping the frequency of audits reasonably high.

The validity of audit as a measure of quality of care will depend both on the criteria used to define good care and the way in which audit is carried out. We have already pointed out that the vagaries of different auditors may wreck audit as a formal method of evaluation. The validity of audit will also be reduced if students prepare sets of notes especially for audit because we do not then know whether they 'care' for their other patients in the same way. But if students and teachers both play their parts properly then the validity of using and auditing problem orientated medical records is beyond question. It encourages and enables students to simulate real clinical practice and it allows teachers to review and comment upon their performance.

CONTINUING EDUCATION

A medical school may consider its work done when its students graduate and begin their work as doctors. But it will have failed them if they do not leave medical school willing and able to learn for the remainder of their professional lives. Doctors must always be prepared to deal with problems which they have not met before and about which they know little. They must learn to apply advances in medical knowledge to the handling of familiar conditions; and they must be able to adapt to new patterns of practice and to the changing expectations of their patients.

The need for continuing education is widely recognised and, as a profession, we have tried to meet this need in a number of different ways. We attend ward rounds and clinical meetings, go to lectures or courses, or attend meetings of specialist societies. Such sessions provide valuable opportunities for contact between colleagues. They also have a limited educational value but we doubt whether they have a great effect on the way in which we care for our patients (surely the aim of continuing education). Firstly because the subject matter which can be covered in this way is, for the individual doctor, necessarily limited; secondly because in most of them the audience plays a relatively passive role, thus violating the important principle that learners should be actively involved in the educational process.

We are bombarded with information from other sources. We receive reading material and audio-visual aids, often of high quality, from drug companies and government agencies. We may subscribe to professional journals or buy textbooks. Much of this information is valuable. It may bring our attention to new material or may serve to reinforce facts we have learned previously. But few of us can hoard this knowledge satisfactorily because it is quickly forgotten if we do not use it. It is therefore important that we should learn to seek information when we require it.

The educational requirements of individual doctors must vary widely and any programme of continuing education should take this into account. It should help us to identify our needs and then help us to satisfy them. Another factor, to which we referred earlier in this chapter, should also be taken into account – that ignorance is one of the least important causes of the mistakes which we make in clinical practice. Defects in our behaviour are more important. Thus if we are to improve our standards we must not only identify gaps in our knowledge but we must also become aware of deficiencies in the care we give to our patients and the reasons for them. We need to have our performance evaluated and to receive feedback on it. When feedback is provided to groups (Godber, 1976) or to individuals (McColl, 1976) there is often a dramatic improvement in performance without any other educational effort being necessary. This improvement may not be sustained if feedback is discontinued and some form of ongoing evaluation or 'audit' seems to be essential in many circumstances.

Unfortunately the idea of audit is anathema to many, if not most, doctors. It seems to imply an accountability to outside authority – an accountability which conflicts with their clinical freedom to act independently in the management of their patients. They fear that 'norms' would be based on elitist standards, are unhappy about the kind of people who might be 'chosen' as auditors, and are worried about the uses to which the results of audit would be put (Alment, 1976).

But if audit does improve performance and make a major contribution to the quality of patient care then it is surely sensible that we should try to introduce it in a form which is acceptable to the profession as a whole. The maintenance of high standards is as much in the interests of our profession as it is in those of our patients and our self-respect must be threatened if we fail to take all necessary steps to promote high standards. If audit is valuable we must use it. But we must use it solely for its educational potential; there should be no question of sanctions against those who do less well than their colleagues as sanctions would interfere with its educational use.

The approach we have advocated for undergraduate education seems appropriate for use in the postgraduate field. Doctors could invite colleagues, from their own specialty or from other specialties, to review their handling of patients and to comment on it in a constructive manner. The 'rules' of audit can be clarified in advance. Auditors could be changed if there were any incompatibilities. In hospital practice there is ample precedent for such an approach as more senior doctors have a responsibility to oversee the clinical performance of their juniors; a similar responsibility is implicit in general practice in the relationship between trainer and trainee. But if we are all to continue learning then it would seem reasonable that we should all submit ourselves to some form of peer review. We agree with the Committee on Competence to Practise (Alment, 1976) that it is a necessary part of a doctor's professional responsibility to assess his work regularly with his colleagues.

If we are to review our handling of patients we need to use our clinical records. Their importance for evaluation was acknowledged by Alment's committee but they felt that present records are unsuitable for this purpose. They suggested that medical records should be improved – to facilitate patient management and to permit retrospective review for evaluation and for research. Their working party on medical records commented on the suitability of POMR for each of these purposes.

A number of groups, in hospitals and in general practice, have used audit of POMR in order to evaluate their work. (Mosser, 1973, Tufo et al, 1973, Burger, 1973, Ellinoy et al, 1973, Milhous, 1973, Hawley, Smith and Grant, 1973). Each group believed that the quality of its work improved. Not only was the work of doctors audited but also that of the allied health professionals who worked in the group.

We believe that this approach to clinical practice is continuing education of the best kind. Doctors audit as well as being audited; they are teachers as well as learners. It requires a marked change in attitudes. At present we are understandably reluctant to criticise the professional actions of our peers. We are all familiar with the guilt engendered when we realise that we did not give our patients the best possible care and we know how this guilt is exacerbated when our inadequacies are revealed. We try to avoid exposure and may be aggressive, resentful or argumentative when challenged. However on these occasions we learn; although the experience may be painful we are less likely to make the same mistake again. Unfortunately many of our mistakes go unrecognised and are never corrected. Surely we should make efforts to uncover our defects whether they are defects of knowledge, of skills or of behaviour. We should invite criticism by our colleagues. As Karl Popper (1974) has pointed out: 'These standards of objective truth and criticism may teach him (the individual man) to try again, and to think again; to challenge his own conclusions, and to use his imagination in trying to find whether and where his own conclusions are at fault. They may teach him to apply the method of trial and error in every field, and especially in science; and thus they may teach him how to learn from his mistakes, and how to search for them. These standards may help him to discover how little he knows, and how much there is that he does not know. They may help him to grow in knowledge, and also to realise that he is growing. They may help him to become aware of the fact that he owes his growth to other people's criticisms, and that reasonableness is readiness to listen to criticism.'

If we are to promote Goals 6 and 8 we must encourage such an attitude to criticism. But we will not do so with an educational system in which constructive criticism and feedback from teacher to student or student to teacher are missing and in which knowledge of facts takes precedence over ability and willingness to seek and use them; nor will we do so if teachers' attitudes render students reluctant to admit their ignorance.

Yet, surprisingly, there is little doubt that these defects all exist in current medical education. They are mentioned by all those who have cause to write on the subject and the present system has few if any defenders. We tend to teach as we were taught, we lack feedback on the effects of our teaching and we put more thought into the content of our teaching than into the principles. Rowntree (1974) was right when he wrote '. . . we cannot plead ignorance of how to teach, for psychology has by now offered us far more insights into human learning and development than we are yet using. Nor, surely, can lack of caring account for more than a fraction of the shortfall in education. I suspect the major factor is the mindlessness of education – the failure of people at every level to ask why they are doing what they are doing or to inquire into the consequences.'

ACKNOWLEDGEMENTS

During the last few years we have had many conversations with Larry Weed about medical education and about the broad aspects of medical care. His ideas permeate this chapter although there are only two references to his work. Many of his publications in medical education are listed in the bibliography at the end of this book. They are well worth reading.

We would like to thank the Dean of the Royal Free Hospital School of Medicine, Dr. Bruce MacGillivray, for his permission to present information about recent curricular developments at our Medical School and about results from a survey carried out amongst our medical students. We would also like to thank the teaching staff of the Royal Free Hospital for the time and effort they have expended in implementing the new curriculum. It is only because of their efforts that we can report upon practical experience.

We are indebted to the King Edward's Hospital Fund which has supported us generously since March 1974, and in particular to Sir Francis Avery Jones and Mr. Geoffrey Phalp who have encouraged and sustained our efforts to promote and propagate the Problem Orientated record.

REFERENCES

Adamson, T. E. (1974) The Teaching and Use of the Problem-Oriented Medical Record in Medical Schools, *Journal of Medical Education*, **49**, 905-907.

Alment, E. A. J. (1976) *Competence to Practise*: The Report of a Committee of Enquiry set up for the Medical Profession in the United Kingdom. Copies obtainable from 27 Sussex Place, Regents Park, London NW1 4RG.

Beard, R. (1970) *Teaching and Learning in Higher Education*,. Harmondsworth, Middx.: Penguin.

Benbassat, J. & Schiffman, A., (1976) An Approach to Teaching the Introduction to Clinical Medicine, *Annals of Internal Medicine*, **84**, 477-481.

Burger, C. S. (1973) Audit in a Problem-Oriented Practice. In *Applying the Problem Oriented System*, ed. Walker, H. K., Hurst, J. W. and Woody, M. F. Ch. 8. New York: Medcom Press.

Buzan, A. (1974) *Use Your Head*. London: B.B.C. Publications.

Davies, I. K. (1971) *The Management of Learning*. London: McGraw Hill.

Dearden, G. & Laurillard, D. (1976). *In-Course Assessment of Clinical Performance: A Trial Scheme*. Obtainable at cost from Dr. Neil McIntyre, Academic Department of Medicine, Royal Free Hospital, London N.W.3.

Ellinoy, B. J., Schuster, J. S., Yatsco, J. C. & Rosenthal, L. C. (1973) Pharmacy Audit of Patient Health records - Feasibility and Usefulness of a Drug Surveillance System. In *Applying the Problem Oriented System*, ed. Walker, H. K., Hurst J. W. & Woody, M. F. Ch. 39. New York: Medcom Press.

Elstein, A. S., Kogan, N., Schulman, L. S., Jason, H. & Loupe, M. J. (1972) Methods and Theory in the study of Medical Inquiry, *Journal of Medical Education*, **47**, 85-92.

Enelow, A. J. & Swisher, S. N. (1972) *Interviewing and Patient Care*, New York: Oxford University Press.

Godber, G. (1976) The Confidential Enquiry into Maternal Deaths. A limited study of clinical results. In *A Question of Quality?: Roads to Assurance in Medical Care*, ed. McLachlan, G., pp. 23-33. London: Oxford University Press.

Goldfinger, S. E. & Dineen, J. J. (1977). In *Harrison's Principles of Internal*

Medicine, ed. Thorn, G. W., Adams, R. D., Braunwald, E., Isselbacher, K. J. & Petersdorf, R. G. Ch. 4, pp. 9-12. New York: McGraw-Hill.

Gruver, R. H. & Freis, E. D. (1957) A Study of Diagnostic Errors. *Annals of Internal Medicine,* **47,** No. 108, 108-120.

Guilbert, J.-J. (1976) *Educational Handbook.* Geneva: World Health Organisation.

Hawley, C., Smith, L. & Grant, R. L. (1973) Initiation of an Audit System for Problem Oriented System Psychosocial Care. In *Applying the Problem Oriented System,* ed. Walker, H. K., Hurst, J. W. & Woody, M. F. Ch. 50. New York: Medcom Press.

Hughes, J., Lloyd, G. J. & McIntyre, N. (1978) The quality and Educational Value of Medical Records - A Survey of Student Opinion. *Medical Education.* **12,** 267-272.

Johns, R. J. (1976) In *The Principles and Practice of Medicine* ed. Harvey, A. M., Johns, R. J., Owens, A. H. & Ross, R. S. Ch. 1, pp. 1-6. New York: Appleton Century Croft.

Lloyd, G. J. & Anthony-Samy, B. R. (1977) *Problem Orientated Medical Record: Self-Instructional Manual.* Available from Dr. Neil McIntyre, Academic Department of Medicine, Royal Free Hospital, Pond Street, London N.W.3.

McColl, I. (1976) Observations on the Quality of Surgical Care. In *A Question of Quality?: Roads to Assurance in Medical Care,* ed. McLachlan, G., pp. 49-61. London: Oxford University Press.

McKay, R. J. (1975) In *Nelson Textbook of Pediatrics,* ed. Vaughan, V. C., McKay, R. J., Nelson, W. E. Ch. 5, pp. 221-233. Philadelphia: Saunders.

MacLeod, J. (1976) In *Clinical Examination,* ed. MacLeod, J. Edinburgh: Churchill Livingstone.

Mager, R. F. (1968) *Developing Attitudes Toward Learning,* Belmont, Calif.: Fearon.

Mager, R. F. (1972) *Goal Analysis,* Belmont, Calif: Fearon.

Mager, R. F. (1973) *Measuring Instructional Intent,* Belmont, Calif: Fearon.

Mager, R. F. (1975) *Preparing Instructional Objectives,* Belmont, Calif: Fearon.

Metcalfe, D. H. H., Rector, A. L., Clayden, A. D. & Hallam, L. (1977) *Innovations in Medical Records in the United Kingdom.* King's Fund project paper, No. 16. Obtainable from King's Fund Centre, 126 Albert Street, London NW1 7NF. (Price £1.00).

Milhous, R. L. (1973) The Problem-Oriented Approach to Rehabilitation Medicine. In *Applying the Problem Oriented System,* ed. Walker, H. K. Hurst, J. W. & Woody, M. F. Ch. 42. New York: Medcom Press.

Miller, G. A. (1956) The Magic Number Seven, plus or minus two: some limits on our capacity for processing information, *Psychological Review,* **63,** 81-97.

Miller, G. E., Abrahamson, S., Cohen, I. S., Graser, H. P., Harnack, R. S. & Land, A. (1961) *Teaching and Learning in Medical School,* Cambridge, Mass.: Harvard University Press.

Morgan, W. L. & Engel, G. L. (1969) *The Clinical Approach to the Patient,* Philadelphia: Saunders.

Mosser, R. S. (1973) Education and Quality Control via the Problem Oriented Record. In *Applying the Problem Oriented System,* ed. Walker, H. K., Hurst, J. W. & Woody, M. F. Ch. 36. New York: Medcom Press.

Neelon, F. A. & Ellis, G. J. (1974) *A Syllabus of Problem-Oriented Patient Care,* Boston: Little Brown Co.

Nelson, G. E., Graves, S. M., Holland, R. R., Nelson, J. M., Ratner, J. & Weed, L. L. (1976) *A Performance Based Method of Student Evaluation. Medical Education,* **10,** 33-42.

Parlett, M. & Hamilton, D. (1976) Evaluation as Illumination. In *Curriculum Evaluation Today: Trends and Implications* ed. Tawney, D. Ch. 5, pp. 84-101. London: Macmillan.

Popper, K. R. (1974) *Conjectures and Refutations,* London: Routledge and Kegan Paul.

Prior, J. A. & Silberstein, J. S. (1973) *Physical Diagnosis,* Saint Louis: C. V. Mosby.

Pyke, D. (1976) Sources of Error, *World Medicine*, Jan. 14th, 24.

Robson, J. R. (1973) In *Curriculum Changes in the United Kingdom Medical Schools*. Dundee: Association for the Study of Medical Education.

Rowntree, D. (1974) *Educational Technology in Curriculum Development*, London: Harper & Row.

Tufo, H. M., Eddy, W. M., Van Buren, H. C., Bouchard, R. E., Twitchell, J. C. & Bedard, L. (1973) Audit in a Practice Group. In *Applying the Problem Oriented System*, ed. Walker, H. K., Hurst, J. W. & Woody, M. F. Ch. 4. New York: Medcom Press.

Voytovich, A. E. (1973) Evaluation of a Nonthreatening Audit System in a Large Teaching Hospital. In *Applying the Problem Oriented System*, ed. Walker, H. K., Hurst, J. W. & Woody, M. F. Ch. 29. New York: Medcom Press.

Walker, H. K., Hall, W. D. & Hurst, J. W. (1976) *Clinical Methods: The History, Physical and Laboratory Examinations*, Boston: Butterworths.

Walker, H. K., Hurst, J. W. & Woody, M. F. (1973) *Applying the Problem Oriented System*, New York: Medcom Press.

Weed, L. L. (1968) Medical Records that Guide and Teach, *New England Journal of Medicine*, **278**, 593-600, 652-657.

Weed, L. L. (1969) *Medical Records, Medical Education and Patient Care*, Cleveland, Ohio: Press of Case Western Reserve University.

Whitehead, A. N. (1962) Technical Education and its relation to Science and Literature. In *The Aims of Education and Other Essays*, Ch. 4. London: Ernest Benn.

Computerisation of the problem orientated record

STEPHEN V. CANTRILL, M.D.

Research Associate, PROMIS Laboratory, College of Medicine, University of Vermont, Burlington, Vermont, USA

This chapter describes the goals, principles, and experience of a medical information system based on the Problem Orientated Medical Record. The general problems in the health care system which this system seeks to solve will be discussed. There then will be a short discussion of the reasons so many attempts to solve these problems with computers have failed. This will be followed by a discussion of the development and operation of the Problem Orientated Medical Information System (PROMIS).

CURRENT SYSTEM PROBLEMS IN MEDICINE

It is widely agreed that many problems exist today in the practice of medicine. Four of the most important include:

1. Lack of coordination among those who supply care to an individual
2. Excessive reliance on memory in the delivery of that care both in terms of knowledge of the patient and knowledge of the medical literature
3. Lack of recorded logic of the reasons that observations were made or specific actions taken
4. Lack of feedback loops in medicine which prevent the use of available patient information to improve the care of an individual patient or to do population studies.

Lack of coordination of care

Due largely to the increased complexity of the health care system, a single patient's overall health care is usually poorly coordinated. Coordination was probably easier in the past because health care was frequently provided by a single person – the family doctor. Now our care involves interactions among generalists, specialists, nurses, pharmacists, laboratories, physician's assistants, dieticians, and others, each ostensibly working toward the goal of better health for the patient but each doing so by applying his expertise only to those problems in his bailiwick. Because each is acting on his own, without full knowledge of the actions of others, much work is duplicated or done at cross purposes. Even when providers attempt to communicate about a patient, the results are frequently failures: lost consultation letters, misplaced laboratory results, and disappearing radiology reports which all contribute to chaotic patient care. This problem could be solved by the use of a single health record for each patient throughout his lifetime, accessible only to those involved in the patient's health care.

Reliance on memory

There are two aspects to the problem of reliance on memory in delivering patient care. First, we health care providers try to remember too many facts about our individual patients. This is fostered by problems with the written record: frequently we cannot find the old record, it is incomplete or we do not take the time to sort through it. We may then, for example, inadvertently give the same patient the same medication which had previously caused a bad drug reaction. Second, we rely too much on our memory for medical facts because referring to the literature when necessary 'takes too much time.' Again, this causes errors, for example, prescribing the wrong dose of a medication because we 'remembered' the dosage regimen incorrectly. This problem could be easily solved by a tool which would couple us to up-to-date medical information and patient records as we went about the task of providing patient care.

Lack of preserved logic of delivered care

In the traditional source orientated medical record, little attempt is made to support an explicit linkage between what observations are made of the patient, what assessments are made about the patient, and what actions are taken for the patient. For example, orders are written without any explicit statement of the problem the physician is treating or what he hopes to accomplish with such treatment. Consequently, we cannot reliably reconstruct why we did what we did. Such a record denies us the ability to learn from our past actions or to follow adequately, over time, the course of any single patient's single disease. The health provider, just as the chronic gambler, sees his occasional success as a justification of his behaviour. To avoid this trap of self-delusion, we need a method of organising the record logically in order to communicate better with others and with ourselves.

Lack of effective feedback loops
Feedback is defined as the introduction of part of the output of a system as an input for the purposes of correction and control of the system. Medicine requires feedback at two levels: the care of our individual patients and the overall care of a population of patients. Reviewing our care, through audit of the records of individual patients, enables us to see our own failures as well as successes so that we may readjust our actions, improving performance as we go. For example, if we consistently, but unknowingly, ignore problems which are identified in the Data Base, we could alter our behaviour if we were made aware of our deficiencies. Review of our care of large groups of patients enables us to uncover new correlations between treatments and outcomes, leading to the advancement of the science of medicine. This feedback can occur most effectively if we have a method for recording what we do in an unambiguous, standard way for large numbers of patients.

Current communication tools in medicine, namely the written, source orientated record and oral communication, are inadequate to solve these four problems. The written Problem Orientated Medical Record assists in providing a record of the logic of medical care. The other problems can be solved by a computerised Problem Orientated Medical Information System.

THE FAILURES OF COMPUTERS IN MEDICINE

Computers have been used successfully in specific, limited areas in medicine, such as automated pulmonary function studies, and in the opening of exciting new areas, such as computerised axial tomography, but there has been failure in ordering the relationships of these specific areas to one another in the total care of patients. If the goal is better patient care, it is not enough to computerise the laboratory so we can do 10 times as many haematocrits; we must also know why we are doing so many and what is being done with the results. The solution to the larger system problems in medicine will be difficult to achieve if we continue to neglect the integration of these pieces. This integration can be accomplished by having medical personnel work directly with patient data and up-to-date medical information through on-line computer terminals. This requires a structured, integrated approach based on a reliable computer system.

Lack of reliable computer systems has been a major shortcoming in computer applications in medicine. A system, to be trusted and therefore used, *must* be reliable. Periods of unavailability must be non-existent or very limited. Also, it must not lose patient information entrusted to it. These capabilities have not often been achieved.

An additional shortcoming has been lack of system responsiveness. A system, to be usable, must respond quickly to the user's request for information; to prevent frustration it must keep up with the user's mind. Most forms of human-computer communication, such as typewriters and many television-like devices, respond too slowly for user satisfaction.

A further difficulty has been lack of the ability to generalise and keep to an appropriate scale: systems which have been successful in single sites are so specific to the requirements of those sites that they cannot be used equally well elsewhere. It may not be possible to scale down a system designed for a 300 bed hospital for use in a 20 physician group practice. Or, a system which supports 10 computer terminals in a responsive manner, may slow down so much in an application requiring 20 computer terminals that its performance is no longer acceptable.

A discussion of failures to utilise a structured, integrated approach can best be presented in terms of the four medical system problem areas mentioned earlier.

Lack of coordination
Most computer applications have done little to improve coordination of care because they have usually been 'kingdom' dependent; they have been designed to solve the problems of a specific department (e.g., clinical laboratory) or administrative area (e.g., admissions) rather than dealing with the larger problem of lack of communication among the departments. These piecemeal solutions are frequently implemented with the promise of 'later expansion to all departments,' but plans for accomplishing this are usually vague. Because of these fuzzy plans, subsequent integration of separate systems is extra-ordinarily difficult, if not impossible.

Reliance on memory
Solutions to this problem have frequently failed due to inadequacies of the human-computer interface. The use of slow typewriter-like devices has forced medical users to wait on the computer. Busy

medical personnel cannot afford this time, so technicians are frequently hired to act as an interface. This prevents the medically qualified person from interacting directly and rapidly either with current medical knowledge or with information about his patients, and thus he cannot reduce his reliance on memory in the delivery of care. The limited storage capacity of a computer system may also preclude showing the medical personnel the appropriate information at the right time. Systems used only for the retrieval of medical facts have often failed because they rely on user initiative; the user determines if, and when, he should turn from his memory to recorded knowledge. Books have failed in the same role, so it is not so surprising that computers would fail also. This inherent deficiency is overcome only by coupling the reference function to the function of actually caring for the patient. This coupling function is the essence of the PROMIS system and will be discussed in detail below.

Lack of preserved logic

Most computer applications do little to preserve the logic of health care because they are based on the traditional source orientated record; its structure is dependent upon the source of the information and it does not demand why information was acquired or how it was used. The logic of care is preserved if the computer system is built around the basic structure of the Problem Orientated Medical Record as information cannot be ordered or reported unless the relevant problems have been identified. (The only exception is information in the Data Base.) Both storage and retrieval of information in a system must adhere to this principle if the logic of care is to be preserved.

Lack of effective feedback loops

Efficient review of individual patient records and groups of records requires the records to be in electronic form, available to the computer. Most computer applications in medicine do not have the capability to keep this amount of information available and are, therefore, unable to even begin solving this problem.

THE PROMIS SYSTEM

The Problem Orientated Medical Information System (PROMIS) was designed to solve the health care problems of coordination, memory, logic and feedback by completely replacing traditional paper records with an electronic problem orientated record which is retrieved and updated directly by medical professionals making choices from words and phrases presented to them on a television-like terminal device.

A prototype PROMIS system was in operation for six months on a general medical ward and for nearly four years on a gynaecology ward in a large teaching hospital. This system supported simultaneous operation of 30 touch-sensitive television-like terminal devices coupled to a single minicomputer (Schultz, Cantrill, Morgan, 1971). More than 3000 patients were cared for using this system during more than four years of its operation. The system is currently being redeveloped with major improvements. The redeveloped system is modular in design, allowing for installations to be scaled to the patient load of a specific institution, clinic or group practice. Installations supporting from 30 to 500 terminals are envisaged.*

The prototype PROMIS system demonstrated solutions to many general problems seen in other computer applications. Through redundant hardware, careful maintenance and good diagnostic tools the system was made to be very reliable, being available to users more than 99.6 per cent of the time, with scheduled 24 hour/day operation. The system was designed to be responsive to facilitate use. The system would commonly respond to a medical user's selection of data from the terminal screen by presenting another screen of information within 600 milliseconds, 50 per cent of the time. This rapid access was to large amounts of information; the patient's complete record was available on the terminal during his hospital stay in addition to the more than 30,000 displays of medical information available for guidance.

The prototype system solved the problem of lack of coordination by allowing access to the electronic record by qualified medical personnel throughout the institution. Terminals on the ward, in the operating suite, in the pharmacy, in the clinical laboratory, and in the department of radiology demonstrated the synergism possible with this coupling. The electronic record became a stronger vehicle for communication among physicians, nurses, pharmacists, radiologists, social workers, and others. In the redeveloped system, we plan to bridge the institutional gap, supplying a single patient record for use wherever the patient receives care.

The problem of reliance on memory was solved by the PROMIS system by having medical professionals use the system directly. The medical user would sit at a TV screen, making appropriate selections by touching the screen from a series of lists presented to him. This facile interface (discussed further below) allowed the professional to interact easily and quickly with

---

*At the time of going to press, the redeveloped system had been in operation for more than 18 additional months on a medical ward, serving more than 1200 additional patients.

1. Data from the patient's record .
2. Information from the current medical literature contained on the more than 30,000 displays which provided guidance to the user.

The currency and correctness of these displays were maintained through elaborate audit and review protocols involving outside experts and library personnel.

The prototype PROMIS system guaranteed preservation of medical logic because all care was problem orientated. But this did not mean lack of flexibility in retrieval. Due to the ease of manipulating data in electronic form, patient information could be retrieved by problem, by chronology across all problems, and by source (e.g., laboratory, radiology). This preservation of logic and flexibility of retrieval also facilitated audit and review of patient records (Nelson *et al*, 1976).

Use of the computer terminal
The computer terminal was quite easy for medical professionals to use (Fig. 6.1). As mentioned, the terminal was a television-like device. It could display 1000 characters of information in 20 lines of 50 characters each and had 20 touch-sensitive fields. A user was confronted with a display containing choices of different (appropriate) words or phrases; he then selected the appropriate choice for his purpose by touching the screen at the position of that choice. The terminal sensed the touch and transmitted a signal to the central processing unit (computer) where information in the display from which the selection was made and the position of the user's touch on the screen would be processed to determine what to display next. The next display might be a fixed set of choices or might contain patient data. Figure 6.2 is a short example of a series of displays one might see during the entry of part of a present illness on 'depression.'

Both fixed displays and patient data were stored on rotating disks (mass memory) and brought into the central processing unit on demand to be transmitted to a user sitting at his terminal. When the user reached a point in his interaction where he needed to store data into the patient record, he inspected and confirmed all the data he had generated by his selections and the computer updated the patient record accordingly.

For those medical content areas where the displays were not complete or a rare finding required description, the medical user could enter free form data by typing in via a keyboard attached to the terminal. Less than one per cent of all data were typed in, more than 99 per cent being entered via the branched-logic displays. All typed-in data were captured and could be analyzed and used to help update the medical content displays.

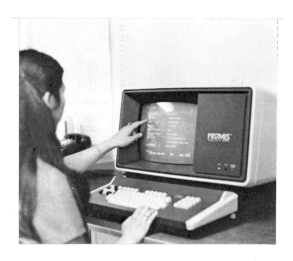

Fig. 6.1 Touch sensitive terminal used for storage and retrieval of patient records in the PROMIS system.

Confidentiality of patient information was guarded by requiring each user to enter a password which allowed him access to the system and identified him as the author of all data which he was to enter. Access to specific patient records and to specific portions of a record was limited by the user's class (physician, laboratory technician, etc.) and by the location of his terminal (ward, laboratory, radiology, etc.). In more than four years of operation, there were no known violations of system confidentiality.

PROMIS IN OPERATION – INTERACTIONS WITH PATIENT RECORDS

When the medical professional sat down to use the terminal, he first chose the patient, whose record he was to interact with, from a list of patients on his ward or service presented on his terminal screen. Having chosen a patient, he was enabled to select any of the four phases of medical action – the Data Base, Problem Formulation, Initial Plans, and Progress Notes – in order to add to or retrieve from that part of his patient's record. The following describes how this might be done.

Data base

The nurse entered the patient's chief complaint, patient profile and the general appearance and vital signs components of the physical examination. The patient, after only two to four minutes of instruction, entered her own review of systems by answering a series of up to 275 yes/no and multiple choice questions. Only the positive responses were stored in the record. (Questionnaires could be displayed in Spanish as well as English, with the English translation stored in the record.) The Review of Systems was then retrieved and reviewed by medical students and house officers. Positive responses were developed into present illnesses by touching selections in branched-logic displays specific for each symptom (Fig. 6.2). The displays used to define present illnesses were built by physicians and approved by expert subspecialists, as were all medical content displays in the system. This allowed any thorough and reliable person with

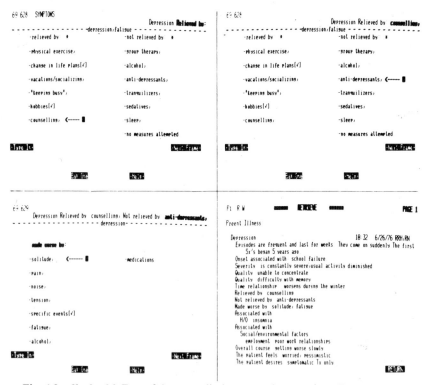

Fig. 6.2a, 2b, 2c, 2d Four of the many displays seen when entering a Present Illness on the symptom 'depression.' The arrow and block indicate the selection made by the user to take him to the next display in the sequence. Note data being entered into record on top of dashed line. Bottom right (6.2d) the completed Present Illness as it exists in the patient's record.

some medical training to gather present illnesses, freeing the physician for more complex tasks. The physical examination would then be entered in a similar manner using up to 1410 branching displays.

Problem formulation

After completion of the Data Base, the physician formulated the patient's problems by making a series of selections on displays. A problem would be stated at its level of definition, ranging from a symptom to a firm diagnosis. The displays facilitated further description of problems by serving to guide the user, frequently providing him with criteria to help him use consistently precise language. These criteria or definitions were derived from the literature with the citation noted on the display (Fig. 6.3). Attached to each problem statement, though not apparent to the user, was an internal code number which was used by the system to expedite access to plans appropriate to that specific problem statement.

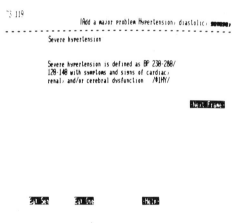

Fig. 6.3 An example of a display defining the term 'severe' as a descriptor for 'Hypertension, diastolic.' The '/ 1HY/' is a reference to a literature citation available to the user upon request.

The system facilitated easy updating of any problem when new information gave added insight. Problems could be added or their status changed (e.g. from active to inactive) at any time. An example of a problem list from a patient on the gynaecology service is shown in Figure 6.4.

Initial plans and other plans

Initial plans were entered for appropriate problems. The physician selected each problem for which he wished to enter an Initial Plan from the list of that patient's problems. (Plans under Progress Notes

```
 - - - - - - - - - - - - - Total Problems - - - - - - - - - - - - - - - - -
 1  Ascites by history (1973) -> Res/Inact                         7/82/74

 2  Adenoca-Corpus Uteri stage not specified                      7/82/74
    ->Adenoca-Corpus Uteri stage IB-g1                             7/85/74
    ->Total hysterectomy w/ bilateral salpingoooophorectomy w/ incidental
      appendectomy for adenoca-corpus uteri                       7/17/74

 3  Anemia, chronic, normocytic, normochromic                     7/82/74

 4  Azotemia (1973) -> Res/Inact                                  7/82/74

 5  Pelvic mass documented by X-ray [IVP]                         7/82/74

 6  Primary hypothyroidism                                        7/82/74

 7  [Rt thigh numbness and paresis] by history                   7/82/74

 8  Systolic murmur [functional]                                  7/82/74
                                                              -More Ques-
```

Fig. 6.4 An example of a patient Problem List from a patient on the Gynaecology service. 'Res/Inact' means resolved or inactivated. Brackets enclose typed-in information.

were also entered in this manner. This description applies to both.) The 'Plans' selection allowed the medical user to

1. Gather additional information to help assess a problem
2. Gather data to rule out specific entities possibly causing the problem
3. Gather information to assist in managing a problem
4. Order treatment for the problem
5. Order patient education.

Each of these components of the plan was individualised for many problems in the system. For example, for the problem of 'Hypertension, diastolic, mild' the system contained displays based on the current literature tailored for each of the first four sections of the plans, detailing how to work-up, treat and follow this problem. These displays removed reliance on memory and allowed a new intern to work-up this problem with a degree of accuracy and completeness comparable to a subspecialist. These displays did not constrain the user; he was free to order whatever he pleased – but the displays served to guide him. It is important to note that the presentation of this disease and patient-specific data to the user is not dependent upon the user's initiative, but rather a natural process of making selections from the presented displays. More than 700 specific disease entities have some degree of problem-specific information in the system. There is certainly much more information to programme into the system, but we feel that the prototype system adequately demonstrated the validity of this approach.

This access to the most up-to-date information from the medical literature, coupled with the instant access to specific data concerning the patient under consideration, facilitates good care flowing from the integration of these two sources of knowledge. Good care requires the integration of patient information with large quantities of known medical facts; paper methods to assist in this process, such as paper-based algorithms, are unmanageable if they contain the required degree of detail. The PROMIS system, however, supplies the user with rapid and reliable access to thousands of appropriate displays without confusion or frustration.

Having this problem-specific information available and up-to-date places great responsibility on a system. Ideally, this content would be maintained by a national or international group who could draw on the best experts in every field to create, maintain, audit, and validate displays in their area of expertise. Since such a group could not be started, we undertook the task ourselves. The creation and maintenance of the displays was done by a small group of physicians and library science personnel. The auditing and validation was done by recognised outside experts (Gustafson et al 1977).

Progress notes

All notes written about any problem after the Initial Plan for that problem were considered Progress Notes. This included physician's notes and nurse's notes. All Progress Notes were entered by first selecting the appropriate problem on the terminal screen from the patient's list of problems. Physicians and nurses then entered 'Symptomatic,' 'Objective,' 'Assessment' or 'Plans' information. The Symptomatic and Objective selections took the user to frames specific for the body system of the problem. The Plans section was entered as described above in 'Initial Plans.'

Nurses were encouraged to enter Progress Notes according to the severity and rate of change of each problem of each patient under their care. They used the same displays as the physician, although some displays were used more by nurses than by physicians.

Operative notes, radiology reports, clinical laboratory reports, social service consultations, specialist consultations were also entered as Progress Notes under the problem they pertained to.

Data retrieval

The above four sections comprise the basic patient record. This data was kept in electronic form in the computer system during a patient's hospital course; there were no written records maintained in parallel. Patient information could be retrieved at any time at any terminal by an appropriately identified medical user. Since the record was in electronic form, data could be retrieved from it in many different ways. Information could be retrieved on a specific problem, on all problems chronologically, or in flowsheet format. Current outstanding drug orders, investigations and accumulated charges were also available by problem. The problem of absent or lost records was non-existent. Any number of users could simultaneously retrieve from or add to a record.

We have discussed entry and retrieval of data of patient care based on the structure of the Problem Orientated Record. This generated record serves as a nucleus for a total system, the additional components of which will now be discussed.

Ward operations

1. Nurses used the system to enter all nurse-related patient data. As noted above, there were no separate nurses' notes, but rather all nurses entered progress notes on patient's problems using the same displays as physicians. Thus, notes of little value ('patient apparently slept well') had been replaced with data about the patient's progress in a problem orientated fashion.

2. Because access to records at any time could be guaranteed, all nurses as a group reviewed the last 24 hours of progress on each patient on the ward at each change of shift. This was a dramatic departure from the traditional, anecdotal, hit-or-miss nurse's report.

3. Most orders were transmitted automatically to the appropriate ancillary area (e.g., pharmacy). The nurse was notified automatically that the order was written but no further effort on her part was required to route the order. Lists of pending drug orders, laboratory tests, radiology studies and nursing procedures were available to nurses for all patients on the nursing unit. These lists were available on paper and on the terminal screen. This capability replaced the major functions of the nursing Kardex with a dynamic list which required little nursing effort to keep it up-to-date.

4. Nursing procedures were entered into the system for reference in the delivery of nursing care. Previously, these procedures were open to interpretation because of the difficulty in updating and maintaining easily accessible documentation of each procedure. Entry of these procedures into the system forced an explicitness and a standardisation which encouraged discussion and resolution of disagreement about each procedure (Gane, 1976).

Pharmacy

Orders for drugs were automatically transmitted to the pharmacy. As a result of the branching-logic of all ordering sequences, all drug orders contained complete drug name, route, dose, frequency and duration of order. The order transmitted to the pharmacy also included the problem under which the drug was ordered and identification of the ordering physician. Simultaneously, if the drug had been deemed potentially dangerous for patient use (and most were), it was placed on a list of drug orders to be reviewed by the pharmacist. The pharmacist was required to review that patient's current problem list (with special attention to the problem for which the drug was ordered), that patient's list of outstanding drug orders, and the information contained in the following categories in the system for the specific drug: 'Check Problem List For;' 'Side Effects To Watch For;' 'Drug Interactions (antagonises, antagonised by, potentiates, potentiated by);' 'Test Interactions;' and 'Usual Dose' (Nelson, 1972). Armed with patient-specific and drug-specific information viewed at a terminal in the pharmacy, the pharmacist consulted with the unit nurse or ordering physician if he felt the drug order should be altered for maximum patient benefit. During one study, this was indicated in 11 per cent of drugs ordered. Such a patient orientated drug review was possible only because the pharmacist was coupled to the actual patient record which, because it was problem orientated, linked each drug to a particular problem.

The pharmacist also used his terminal in the dispensing of medications for the nursing unit. The list of outstanding drugs for each patient on the ward was retrieved to the terminal screen and used as a guide for filling patient Unit Dose drug transport containers. The Unit Dose drug distribution system was initiated at the hospital as a result of the installation of PROMIS in the pharmacy.

The computer system was, of course, used by the nursing staff to chart medications given to patients. This data, as well as summary statistics by drug of how many doses were dispensed over a period of time with accumulated dollar value, were available for review by the pharmacist. PROMIS can serve as an inventory control system, a charge center income accumulation system and a tool for reviewing prescription trends in an institution.

Radiology
The radiologist was also coupled to the patient record. Requests for radiology studies were transmitted automatically to the department of radiology in the form of:

1. patient-identifying information
2. the problem for which the study was requested
3. what entities, if any, the clinician was trying to implicate by the study (e.g., R/O TBC)

4. the study requested
5. the physician who requested it
6. a complete list of the patient's problems.

After the study had been done, the radiologist entered his report in the patient's record under the problem for which the study was ordered through a series of branched-logic displays on the terminal. The radiologist had access to the patient's entire medical record via his terminal whenever he felt he needed additional clinical information.

As soon as the radiologist confirmed his report, it was available in the patient's electronic record throughout the system. As an example, it was not uncommon to have a patient leave the nursing unit at 8:30 a.m. to go for a barium meal, with the subsequent report available in the record by 10:30 a.m. that same day.

The radiologist also had access to all outstanding radiology orders for the nursing unit. This list, available on the terminal at any time, was valuable in identifying studies not done which should have been done and studies done but misplaced and therefore not reported.

Administrative reports detailing the numbers of the different studies done in the radiology department, valuable for both long-term department planning and short-term department management, were generated.

Clinical laboratory

Although integration with the clinical laboratory was not complete before redevelopment began, most laboratory data were entered directly by personnel in the laboratory. Most of the laboratory data from the morning blood drawings were available in the patient's electronic record by 11:30 a.m. As with radiology, the laboratory knew for what problem a study was ordered. The laboratory also had access to a list of pending requests. Draw lists and work lists, while not feasible for a single nursing unit, could be generated for the entire institution. Statistical summaries of numbers ordered and reported were also available.

Fiscal information

A direct result of work done to automate the patient's record was the automatic generation of a Problem Orientated List of Charges, an example of which is shown in Figure 6.5. Since the record contained the history of all services rendered to the patient on a problem basis, it required only the step of assigning each service a charge value, and then summing those values by charge area (pharmacy, radiology, etc.) by problem. These charges were based on what was actually done for the patient, rather than, less reliably, what was ordered to be done. For institutions charging on a per-service basis, it would be a small step to convert the List of Charges to an actual bill. The List of Charges could be retrieved on an available terminal screen for any patient. It was always completely up-to-date. This mechanism could supply feedback to the physician as to incurred charges for a single patient, as well as, over a long term, supplying necessary data to allow valid cost-benefit evaluation of different modes of care in the population.

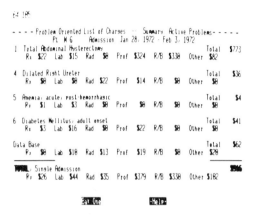

Fig. 6.5 A prototype of a Problem Orientated List of Charges, using data captured by the PROMIS system. This is a summary list. A more detailed list could also be produced for administrative/billing purposes. 'Rx' = pharmacy charges, 'Lab' = clinical laboratory, 'Rad' = radiology, 'Prof' = professional fee (including that from clinical laboratory and radiology), 'R/B' = room and board, 'Other' includes operating room charges, anaesthesiology charges, etc.

Ambulatory care

Although the PROMIS system has been used primarily in a hospital setting, extension of the system to include ambulatory care should present no major medical or technical problems. Medically, the system is not limited to specialised problem areas, but rather, is capable of covering the full range of problems encountered in a general practice, including psychiatric, social and demographic problems. Most of the medical content in the system is appropriate for outpatient as well as inpatient care. The system facilitates dealing with ambulatory patients by allowing for definition, management and follow-up of 'Temporary Problems,' problems felt to be of acute, self-limited nature which do not require detailed management or follow-up (e.g. an uncomplicated upper respiratory tract infection). This division of the Problem List into 'Temporary' and 'Permanent' problems allows all illnesses to be followed in a problem orientated fashion, but allows easy separation of the chronic or severe problems from the relatively minor, short-lived problems.

Technically, minor difficulties may develop with the extension of the PROMIS system to ambulatory care in the amount of computer (mass memory) storage required because of the greater number of patients seen in ambulatory care as opposed to inpatient care. These problems are not felt to be insurmountable at this time.

User acceptance

During the more than four years of operation, the PROMIS system was used by more than 500 individuals as the sole mechanism to retrieve and add information in patient records. Included were physicians, nurses, medical students, house staff, radiologists, pharmacists, social workers, ward secretaries, dieticians and laboratory technicians. Most of these users required less than a few hours instruction to be able to use the system well. The system had nearly unanimous acceptance from all classes of users, with the exception of physicians and house staff, who were, as a group, ambivalent about the system, but who did use it. Those who had increased opportunity to relate their professional skills to the care of patients through the PROMIS system were most enthusiastic about using the system.

Nurses, by and large, used the system very well and were quick to realise its power and potential. Because the system could move information at the speed of light and because that information was structured, with the logic of the author preserved, nurses became an informed participant in a team effort; they no longer had to carry out orders without knowing why. For example, for a patient who went to surgery, the nurse had access to the complete operative report, including all post-operative orders, by problem, before the patient left the operating suite, which allowed her to make more accurate and meaningful observations of patient progress and the effects of therapy.

Pharmacists also accepted the system wholeheartedly. Automatic transmission of the complete, legible drug order to the pharmacy with the statement of the problem for which the drug was ordered allowed them to do much more than be purely mindless dispensers of medication. The problem orientated order and the rapid access the pharmacists had to the patient's record via their terminal and to current drug information in the medical content displays allowed them to act in a professional advisory role to help ensure that the patients got the best possible drug therapy.

While most other personnel accepted the system with enthusiasm, the greatest diversity of acceptance was among the physicians and house staff. This is understandable since the PROMIS system represents a discontinuity with respect to the traditional practice of medicine. The PROMIS system promulgates rules and standards in terms of completeness and disciplined medical action whereas the traditional system allowed each practitioner to make up his own rules and change them at will. The system also acts as a strong unifying factor among all medical personnel dealing with a single patient, making it possible for each to know what the other is doing for the patient and why he is doing it. Some specialists, who were not accustomed to caring for the patient's problem in their area of expertise in the context of the rest of the patient's problems, found this explicitness difficult to accept because it left them open to questions from other professional personnel as to why they took a certain action. Most physicians are not used to having their actions questioned.

The PROMIS system was also threatening to those individuals who traded heavily on their own memories in the delivery of care. They were offended by the implication that they could not remember all that was required to deliver good care to patients.

Many physicians, however, were enthusiastic about using the PROMIS system. They appreciated and gladly followed the medical content guidance supplied by the system. They understood the necessity of a defined Data Base and liked the fact that the patient herself and other ancillary personnel could be utilised to gather much of it. They also appreciated the reliable, rapid reporting of laboratory and radiology results directly into the patient's record and the ability to retrieve any part of the record from any terminal at any time. The use of the PROMIS system for more than four years clearly demonstrated that many physicians are willing to use this system for patient care.

Cost of the PROMIS system

If any computer system is to be widely used, it must be economically feasible. We feel that the PROMIS system fulfils this requirement. Current costs of a complete PROMIS system are difficult to compute for such reasons as the continuing precipitous decline in the cost of minicomputer hardware and the unknown economies of scale of installing several similar systems; however, a gross cost of approximately five dollars per bed day has been estimated. The net cost of such a system, however, may well be a savings for the health care system as a whole. Savings could be anticipated through elimination of repeat radiology and laboratory studies due to lost reports, decreased length of stay due to elimination of these repeat studies and possibly fewer severe drug reactions and fewer total visits because a single record facilitates coordinating resources, allowing the most to be done for a patient during each visit. It may be truly false economy to continue with our current chaotic system for communicating in health care, when for a relatively small sum, we can solve so many problems that obstruct good care.

REQUIREMENTS FOR SUCCESS OF THIS SYSTEM

The PROMIS system described here has demonstrated solutions to major problems in the practice of medicine. If one agrees that an appropriate goal is the solution of the health care problems of lack of coordination, reliance on memory, lack of preserved logic and inadequate feedback loops, then this system must be viewed as viable and desirable. Success in the use of the PROMIS system requires commitment at an institutional level to solve these problems in medicine. Each of these problems, in turn, presents specific requirements if the system is to be used most effectively.

The PROMIS system, through its requirements for explicitness and its coupling capability, not only points out those areas which require coordination and teamwork between health care personnel but also reveals where such teamwork is not present. For example, explicit plans made by the physician and the nurse may be contradictory. These contradictory plans are not the result of using the PROMIS system; they have been occurring all along, but they have never before been made explicit. To make the best use of the potential coordination requires all professional personnel to be willing to work together as a team, to integrate their combined efforts for the best care of the patient.

For the PROMIS system to be successful at removing the reliance on memory, it must contain vast amounts of information from the medical literature which can be coupled to the user in a useful manner in the context of the specific patients under his treatment. This requires manpower and organisation to update, verify and maintain information contained in the medical content displays. This 'Library of Displays' function, while being a large task, may in fact allow us to save time over the long run by making our efforts to catalogue and file new medical information more cumulative, with greater effect on the actual practice of medicine. Also, if the PROMIS system is properly maintained, it may provide a desirable alternative, with manpower savings, for the current expensive approaches to both graduate and postgraduate medical education.

For the information generated through use of the PROMIS system to be most valuable to the practice of medicine, it must be analysed to detect problems in the delivery of care both at an individual patient level and the population group level. Once these individual and system problems have been detected, leadership must be exercised to use these data to influence and improve care for patients by altering the behaviour of deficient health care providers and correcting those problems in the system itself.

The PROMIS system described here is a tool which permits us to operate within a defined structure with up-to-date medical information whereby we can grow wiser from what we do. The degree to which we will be successful in using the tool to practise 'better' medicine depends upon how we define our goals, set our priorities and how those in positions of medical leadership act to correct deficiencies uncovered by use of the PROMIS system.

ACKNOWLEDGEMENT

This chapter describes the operation of a prototype Computerised Problem Oriented Medical Information System which was in operation for more than four years (1970-1974) at the Medical Centre Hospital of Vermont in Burlington, Vermont, USA. What is described here is not the work of any single individual, but a synergistic effort by computer scientists, physicians, nurses, pharmacists, radiologists, library science personnel, and others under the guidance of Lawrence L. Weed, MD to establish an improved system for the delivery of health care. The work described here was done under a research grant from the United States Department of Health, Education and Welfare, PHS 1 R18 HS 00175 and a grant from the Robert Wood Johnson Foundation.

REFERENCES

Dietrich, P. A. (1973) Problem Oriented Radiology Reporting. In *Applying the Problem Oriented System*, ed. Walker, H. K., Hurst, J. W. & Woody, M. F. Ch. 40, pp. 372-379. New York City: MEDCOM Press.

Gane, D. (1976) An Example of the Effects of Computer Usage on Nursing Practice. In *Your Health Care and How To Manage It*, by Weed, L. L. Ch. 21, pp. 99-106. Essex Junction, Vt., USA: Essex Publishing Co., Inc.

Gilroy, G., Ellinoy, B. J., Nelson, G. E. & Cantrill, S. V. (1977) Integration of Pharmacy into the Computerized Problem-Oriented Medical Information System (PROMIS) - A Demonstration Project. *American Journal of Hospital Pharmacy*, **38**, 155-162.

Gustafson, J. C., Nelson, J. M. & Buller, A. C. (1977) Coordination Medical Literature with Patient Care. *Methods of Information in Medicine*, **16**, 234-240.

Nelson, G. E. (1972) The Problem Oriented Medical Record and Teaching of Clinical Pharmacology. 1 The Journal of Clinical Pharmacology, **12**, 375-381.

Nelson, G. E., Graves, S. M., Holland, R. R., Nelson, J. M., Ratner, J. & Weed, L. L. (1976) A Performance-Based Method of Student Evaluation. *Medical Education*, **10**, 33-42.

Schultz, J. R., Cantrill, S. V. & Morgan, K. G. (1971) An Initial Operational Problem Oriented Medical Record System - For Storage, Manipulation and Retrieval of Medical Data. *Proceedings of the American Federation of Information Processing Societies*, **38**, 239-264.

Schultz, J. R. (1974) An Implementation Independent Description of a Problem Oriented Medical Information System: Philosophical principles and how they are used to Define Technological Goals. *Proceedings of Comcon.* **74**, 179-184.

Weed, L. L. (1976) *Your Health Care and How to Manage it*. Essex Junction, Vt., USA: Essex Publishing Co., Inc.

Weed, L. L., Weed, L. B., Nelson, G. E. & Dietrich, P. A. (1972) Background Paper for Concept of National Library of Displays. In *The Problem Oriented System*, ed. Hurst, J. W. & Walker, H. K. Ch. 29, pp. 258–267. New York City: MEDCOM Press.

Bibliography

References are in chronological order.

Weed, L. L. (1969) *Medical Records, Medical Education and Patient Care,* Cleveland: The Press of the Case Western Reserve University.

Bjorn, J. & Cross, H. (1970) *The Problem-Oriented Private Practice of Medicine - A System for Comprehensive Health Care,* Chicago: Modern Hospital Press.

Hurst, J. W. & Walker, H. K. (1972) eds. *The Problem-Oriented System,* New York: Medcom Press.

Walker, H. K., Hurst, J. W. & Woody, M. F. (1973) eds. *Applying the Problem-Oriented System,* New York: Medcom Press.

Atwood, J. & Yarnall, S. (1974) eds. The Problem-Oriented Record, Special Edition of *The Nursing Clinics of North America,* **Vol. 9,** No. 2, June, Philadelphia: W. B. Saunders Company.

Berni, R. & Readey, H. (1974) *Problem-Oriented Medical Record Implementation, Allied Health Peer Review,* St. Louis: C. V. Mosby Company.

Easton, R. R. (1974) *Problem-Oriented Medical Record Concepts,* New York: Appleton-Century-Crofts.

Mazur, W. P. (1974) *The Problem-Oriented System in the Psychiatric Hospital,* Trainex Medcom Press.

National League for Nursing, (1974) *The Problem-Oriented System - A Multidisciplinary Approach,* Pub. No. 20-1546.

Neelon, F. A. & Ellis, G. J. (1974) *A Syllabus of Problem-Oriented Patient Care,* Boston: Little Brown Co.

Ryback, R. (1974) *The Problem Oriented Record in Psychiatry and Mental Health Care,* New York: Grune and Stratton Inc.

Sandlow, L. J., Hammett, W. J., & Bashook, P. G. (1974) *Problem-Oriented Medical Records. Guidelines for Format and Forms,* Chicago: Michael Reese Medical Center.

Wooley, *et al.* (1974) *Problem Oriented Nursing,* New York: Springer Publishing Co.

Weed, L. L. (1975) *Your Health Care and How to Manage It,* Essex Junction, Vermont: Essex Publishing Co.

National League for Nursing, (1975), The Problem-Oriented System in a Home Health Agency - A Training Manual, *League Exchange,* No. 13. Pub. No. 21-1554.

The College of Family Physicians of Canada, (1977), *Manual for the College Office Record.*

OTHER WRITINGS BY LARRY WEED

Weed, L. L. (1964), Medical Records, Patient Care and Medical Education, *Irish Journal of Medical Science,* **6,** 271-282.

Weed, L. L. (1967), A New Approach to Medical Teaching: Use of the Hospital Record, *Resident Physician,* **13,** 77-93.

Weed, L. L. (1967), *The Patient's Record as an Extension of the Basic Science Training of the Physician*, Case Western Reserve Publication.

Weed, L. L. (1968), Medical Records that Guide and Teach, *New England Journal of Medicine*, **278**, 593–600, 652–657.

Weed, L. L. (1968), What Physicians Worry About: How to Organise Care of Multiple Problem Patients, *Modern Hospital*, **110**, 90–94.

Weed, L. L. (1970), Technology is a Link, Not a Barrier, for Doctor and Patient, *Modern Hospital*, **114**, 80–83.

Weed, L. L. (1971), Quality Control and the Medical Record, *Archives of Internal Medicine*,**127**, 101–105.

Weed, L. L. (1971), The Problem-Oriented Record as a Basic Tool in Medical Education, Patient Care and Clinical Research, *Annals of Clinical Research*, **3**, 131–134.

Weed, L. L. (1971), C.P.C.'s as Educational Instruments, *The New England Journal of Medicine*, **285**, 115–118.

Weed, L. L. (1974), A Touchstone for Medical Education, *Harvard Alumni Bulletin*, November/December, 13–18.

Weed, L. L. (1975), The Problem-Oriented Record – Its Organising Principles and Its Structure, *League Exchange*, **103**, 3–6.

Weed, L. L. (1976), A New Paradigm for Medical Education. In *Recent Trends in Medical Education*, ed. E. F. Purcell. New York: Josiah Macy, Jr. Foundation, pp. 55–93.

Weed, L. L. (1977), The Expectation-Delivery Gap, *Journal of Oklahoma State Medical Association*, **70**, 12–15.

GENERAL

Krismer, J. R. & Cordes, J. F. (1970) Problem-Orientated Record Begins with Patient, *Modern Hospital*, **115**, 81–84.

Dreyfus, E. G. *et al* (1971) Internal Chart Audits in a Neighborhood Health Program: a Problem-oriented Approach, *Medical Care*, **9**, 449–454.

Graves, S. (1971) Better Records: First Step to Better Quality, *Modern Hospital*, **116**, 105–108.

Hurst, J. W. (1971) The Art and Science of Presenting a Patient's Problems, *Archives of Internal Medicine*, **128**, 463–465.

Hurst, J. W. (1971) The Problem-Oriented Record and the Measurement of Excellence, *Archives of Internal Medicine*, **128**, 818–819.

Hurst, J. W. (1971) How to Implement the Weed System, *Archives of Internal Medicine*, **128**, 456–462.

Hurst, J. W. (1971) Ten Reasons Why Weed is Right,·*New England Journal of Medicine*, **284**, 1.

McCanse, A. (1971) Weed's Seed: Problem-Oriented Medical Record, *Missouri Medicine*, **68**, 401.

O'Connor, F. J. (1971) Community Hospital Problem-Oriented Medical Care Service, *Journal of the Maine Medical Association*, **62**, 177.

P.O.M.R. (1971) A Special Collection of Selected Articles, *Medical Record News*, **42**, 29–60.

Tufo, H. M. & Speidel, J. J. (1971) Problems with Medical Records, *Medical Care*, **9**, 509–517.

Benage, J. F. (1972) Problem Oriented Chart, *Journal of the Kansas Medical Society*, **73**, 361–362.

Bryan, T. & Summers, R. W. (1972) How to start using the problem oriented medical record, *Journal of the Iowa Medical Society*, **62**, 183–186.

Fabb, W. (1972) Why A Problem-Oriented Medical Record?, *Medical Practice Management*, **1**, 23–24.

Gardner, L. B. (1972) The Problem-Oriented Record in Critical Care Medicine, *Chest*, **62**, Supplement (pt 2) 63s–69s.

Hurst, J. W., Walker, H. K., & Hall, W. D. (1972) More Reasons why Weed is Right, *New England Journal of Medicine*, **288**, 629–630.

Jervey, A. J. (1972) On the Use of Problem-Oriented Medical Records, *Alaska Medicine*, **14**, 59–61.

(1972) Problem-Oriented Medical Records, (Editorial) *The Lancet*, Feb. 5th.

McIntyre, N., Day, R. C. & Pearson, A. J. G. (1972) Can We Write Better Notes? An Introduction to P.O.M.R. (The Weed Approach), *British Journal of Hospital Medicine*, 603–611.

Weiss, J. J. & Yanez, J. (1972) Our Experience Using Problem-Oriented Records, *Resident Staff Physician*, **18**, 36.

Aronson, M. D. (1973) The Problem-Oriented Record: Two Column Modification, *Journal of the American Medical Association*, **255**, 716.

Bonner, B. B. (1973) Problem-Oriented Medical Records, *Health and Social Service Journal*, 373–374.

Boyle, C. M., Alexander, W. D. & Stevenson, J. G. (1973) A New Hospital Letter for the Specialist Clinic, *Lancet*, 249–251.

Feinstein, A. R. (1973) The Problems of the Problem-Oriented Medical Record, *Annals of Internal Medicine*, **78**, 751–762.

Froom, J. (1973) Conversion to Problem-Oriented Records in an Established Practice: A Timed Study, *Annals of Internal Medicine*, **78**, 254–257.

Gledhill, V. X., Mackay, I. R., Mathews, J. D., Strickland, R. G., Stevens, D. P. & Thompson, C. D. (1973) The Problem-Oriented Medical Synopsis – Applications to Patient Care, Education and Research, *Annals of Internal Medicine*, **78**, 685–691.

Goldfinger, S. E. (1973) Problem-Oriented Record: A Critique from a Believer, *New England Journal of Medicine*, **288**, 606–608.

McIntyre, N. (1973) The Problem-Oriented Medical Record, *British Medical Journal*, 598–600.

Shenkin, B. N. & Warner, D. C. (1973) Giving the Patient his Medical Record: A Proposal to Improve the System, *New England Journal of Medicine*, **289**, 688–691.

Stevenson, J. G., Boyle, C. M. & Alexander, W. D. (1973) A New Hospital Discharge Letter, *Lancet*, 928–931.

Cross, H. D. (1974) The Case for Problem-Oriented Medical Records, *British Journal of Hospital Medicine*, **11**, 65–79.

Fletcher, R. H. (1974) Auditing Problem-Oriented Records and Traditional Records: A Controlled Comparison of Speed, Accuracy and Identification of Errors in Medical Care, *New England Journal of Medicine*, **290**, 829–833.

McIntyre, N. (1974) Obtaining Information from Medical Records, *Journal of the Royal College of Physicians*, **8**, 267–275.

Mason, A. M. S. & Simpson, P. (1974) Doctors as Managers, Medical Audit, *Hospital Update*, 779–784.

Newble, D. T. *et al* (1974) Quality Control of Patient Care – The Practical Application of Problem-Oriented Medical Records, *Australian and New Zealand Journal of Medicine*, **4**, 23–28.

Sandlow, L. (1974) The Problem-Oriented Medical Record: Time Saving Aid in Patient Care, *Postgraduate Medicine*, **56**, 163–167.

Valberg, L. (1974) Measurement of Quality Care. The Place of the Problem-Oriented Record and Other Methods of Evaluating Quality of Care in the Hospital Setting, *Annals of the Royal College of Physicians and Surgeons of Canada*, 325–332.

Burchell, K., Barclay, R. & Ryan, M. P. (1975) The Use of the Problem Oriented Medical Record and Feature Cards in Practice Management and Research, *Health Bulletin* (Edinburgh), **33**, 210–213.

Longenecker, D. P. (1975) Coding Diseases and Problems. How and Why You Should Be Using Problem Oriented Medical Records, *Ohio State Medical Journal*, **71**, 386–387.

Manning, P. R. (1975) The Problem-Oriented Record as a Tool in Management, *Clinical Obstetrics and Gynaecology*, **18**, 175–179.

Phillips, D. F. (1975) Some POMR Criticism Clearly Misdirected, *Hospitals*, **49**, 582—61.

Barclay, R., Burchell, K., Gunn, A. A. & Ryan, M. P. (1976) Towards an Integrated Medical Record, *Health Bulletin* (Edinburgh), **18**, 36–43.

Golodetz, A., Ruess, J. & Milhous, R. L. (1976) The Right to Know: Giving the Patient his Medical Record, *Archives of Physical Medicine and Rehabilitation*, **57**, 78-81.

Hammett, W. H., Sandlow, L. J. & Bashook, P. G. (1976) Format Review: Evaluating Implementation of the Problem-Oriented Medical Record, *Medical Care*, **14**, 857-865.

Lambert, R. P. & Mackay, I. R. (1976) A Problem-Orientated Outpatient Record, *Medical Journal of Australia*, **2**, 368-372.

Roger, F. H., Jocs, M. & Haxhe, J. J. (1976) An Interhospital Problem-Oriented and Automated Discharge Summary, *Methods of Information in Medicine*, **15**, 141-144.

Walker, H. K. (1976) The Problem-Oriented Medical System, *Journal of the American Medical Association*, **236**, 2397-2398.

Stevens, D. P., Stagg, R. & Mackay, I. R. (1977) When Hospitalized Patients see their Own Records, *Annals of Internal Medicine*, **86**, 474-477.

GENERAL PRACTICE

Yarnall, S. & Iverson, N. T. (1971) Structured Problem-Oriented Records in Office Practice, *Northwest Medicine*, **70**, 166-167.

Acheson, H. W. K. (1972) The Clinical Record as an Aid to Continuing Education in General Practice: A Medical Self-Audit, *British Journal of Medical Education*, **6**, 26-28.

Cross, H. (1972) Medical Records and Health Care: The Problem-Oriented Medical Record, *Medical Record News*, **43**, 16-27.

Phillips, T. J. (1972) Problem-Oriented Record in General Practice, *Northwest Medicine*, **71**, 279-280.

Tudor, J. M. (1972) Problem-Oriented Method in Family Practice, *Journal of the Arkansas Medical Society*, **68**, 289-293.

Metcalfe, D. H. H. (1973) Problem-Oriented Medical Records, *Practice Team*, **22**, 11-13.

Tait, I. & Stevens, J. (1973) The Problem-Oriented Medical Record in General Practice, *Journal of the Royal College of General Practitioners*, **23**, 311-315.

Williamson, J. D. (1973) Quality Control, Medical Audit and the General Practitioner, *Journal of the Royal College of General Practitioners*, **23**, 697-706.

Clark, E. M. (1974) Disease Coding in a Problem-Oriented General Practice, *Journal of the Royal College of General Practitioners*, **24**, 469-475.

Curtis, P. (1974) Medical Audit in General Practice, *Journal of the Royal College of General Practitioners*, **24**, 607-611.

Dixon-Warren, B. C. (1974) Measurement of Quality Care. The Place of the Problem-Oriented Record and Other Methods of Evaluating the Quality of Care in an Ambulatory Setting. *Annals of the Royal College of Physicians and Surgeons of Canada*, 313-324.

Froom, J. & Farley, E. S. (1974/75) An Integrated System for the Recording and Retrieval of Medical Data in a Primary Care Setting. Part 1. The Age Sex Register, *Journal of Family Practice*, **1**, 44–46. Part 2. Classification of Diseases, *Journal of Family Practice*, **1**, 47–48. Part 3. The Diagnostic index-E Book, *Journal of Family Practice*, **1**, 45–48. Part 4. Family Folders, *Journal of Family Practice*, **1**, 49–51. Part 5. Implications of Filing Charts by Area of Residence, *Journal of Family Practice*, **1**, 43–47. Part 6. The Problem Oriented Medical Record, *Journal of Family Practice*, **1**, 48–51. Part 7. The Encounter Form and the Minimum Basic Data Set, *Journal of Family Practice*, **2**, 37–41. Part 8. The

Individual Patient's Medical Record, *Journal of Family Practice,* **2,** 43–53.

Murray, M., Sydenham, D. & Westlake, R. (1974) A Questionnaire as a Data Base in Problem-Orientated Records, *Journal of the Royal College of General Practitioners,* **24,** 572–575.

Otway, W. (1974) Problem-Orientated Personal (P.O.P.) Medical Records for General Practice, *New Zealand Medical Journal,* 724–726.

Rakel, R. E. (1974) The Problem-Oriented Medical Record (POMR), *American Family Physician,* **10,** 100–111.

Shires, D. B., Rozovsky, L., Cameron, A. G. & Steves, L. C. (1974) Just for the Record: The Problem-Oriented Approach, *Canadian Family Physician,* **20,** 47–50.

West, S. R. (1974) A Comprehensive Data Base in General Practice Records, *New Zealand Medical Journal,* **79,** 721–724.

Widmer, R. B. (1974) Problem-Oriented Medical Records in Ambulatory Care, *Journal of the Arkansas Medical Society,* **71,** 113–124.

Woods, J. O. (1974) Improved Record Keeping in General Practice, *Journal of the Royal College of General Practitioners,* **24,** 865–874.

Curtis, P. (1975) Problem-Oriented Medical Records in General Practice. A Simple Approach, *Update,* **11,** 987–995.

Deming, B. & Kimble, J. J. (1975) Adapting the Individual Problem-Oriented Record for Use with Families, *Hospital and Community Psychiatry,* **26,** 334–335.

Jarvis, D. J. A. (1975) The Problem-Oriented Medical Record in the RACGP Record System, *Australian Family Physician,* **4,** 516–520.

Metcalfe, D. (1975) Problem-Oriented Medical Records in General Practice. A Practical Program. 1. Introduction. *Update,* **11,** 1163–1167. 2. The Background Information List. *Update,* **11,** 1287–1289. 3. The Problem List. *Update,* **12,** 391–395. 4. Plans and Progress Notes. *Update,* **12,** 523–524. 5. Using Problem-Oriented Records. *Update,* **12,** 643–646. 6. Adding to the Problem List. *Update,* **12,** 769–772.

Reed, D. E., Lapenas, C., deVries, J. R., Watterson, S. G. & Caton, R., (1975) Non-Physician Development of Problem Lists from Office Records, *Journal of Family Practice,* **2,** 211–212.

Bentsen, B. G. (1976) The Accuracy of Recording Patient Problems in Family Practice, *Journal of Medical Education,* **51,** 311–316.

Hertz, C. G. & Bernheim, J. W. & Perloff, T. N. (1976) Patient Participation in the Problem-Oriented System: A Health Care Plan, *Medical Care,* **14,** 77–79.

Page, O. C. (1976) The Problem-Oriented Approach to Team Practice. In *The Changing Health Care Team,* eds. S. Yoog & S. Yarnall, Seattle; MCSA. pp. 3–15.

Shaw, S. W. (1976) The Team Approach to Family Practice. In *The Changing Health Care Team,* eds. S. Yoog & S. Yarnall. Seattle; MCSA. pp. 22–26.

Sheldon, M. G. (1976) The Problems of Problem-Oriented Records, *Journal of the Royal College of General Practitioners,* **26,** 437–446.

Warren, M. D. (1976) Medical Records in Family Practice. A Review, *Scandinavian Journal of Social Medicine,* **4**(2), 91–101.

Yarnall, S. R. (1976) The Problem-Oriented Approach – A Sine Qua Non for Audit. In *The Changing Health Care Team,* eds. S. Yoog & S. Yarnall. Seattle; MCSA. pp. 161–165.

Dixon-Warren, B. (1977) Tools for the Job: The POMR in Preventive Medicine, *Canadian Family Physician,* **23,** 718–724.

Grace, N. T., Neal, E. M., Wellock, C. E. & Pile, D. D. (1977) The Family-Oriented Medical Record, *Journal of Family Practice,* **4,** 91–98.

PSYCHIATRY

Grant, R. L. & Maletzky, B. M. (1972) Application of the Weed System to Psychiatric Records, *Psychiatry in Medicine,* **3,** 119–129.

Hayes-Roth, F., Longabaugh, R. & Ryback, R. (1972) The Problem-Oriented Medical Record and Psychiatry, *British Journal of Psychiatry,* **121,** 27–34.

Abrams, R. S. *et al.* (1973) Problem-Oriented Recording of Psychosocial Problems, *Archives of Physical Medicine and Rehabilitation,* **54**, 316–319.

Hood, J. N. (1973) Indicating Levels of Probability in the Problem-Oriented Record, *Hospital and Community Psychiatry,* **24**, 253.

Novello, J. R. (1973) The Problem-Oriented Record in Psychiatry, *Journal of Nervous and Mental Disease,* **156**, 349–353.

Ryback, R. & Gardiner, J. (1973) Problem Formulation: A Problem-Oriented Record, *American Journal of Psychiatry,* **130**, 312–316.

Scales, J. E. & Johnson, M. S. (1973) A Psychiatric POMR for Use By a Multi-Disciplinary Team, *Hospitals and Community Psychiatry,* **26**, 371–373.

Spitzer, R. L. (1973) P.O.M.R.: Some Reservations, *International Journal of Psychiatry,* **11**, 376.

Grant, R. L. (1974) The Problem-Oriented Record – A Tool for Teaching and Evaluation of Learning in the New Psychiatric Curriculum. In *Evaluative Methods in Psychiatric Education,* ed. H. L. Muslin *et al.* Washington; American Psychiatric Association, 185–199.

Fowler, D. R. & Longabaugh, R. (1975) The Problem-Oriented Record. Problem Definition. *Archives of General Psychiatry,* **32**, 831–834.

Gaviria, B., Alvis, J. & Zarour, N. (1976) Changing to Problem-Oriented Methods. Implementation in Psychiatric Institutions, *Journal of Nervous and Mental Disease,* **163**, 124–134.

Klonoff, H. & Cox, B. (1975) A Problem-Oriented System Approach to the Analysis of Treatment Outcome, *American Journal of Psychiatry,* **132**, 836–841.

Liston, E. H. (1976) Use of Problem-Oriented Medical Record in Psychiatry: A Survey of University-Based Residency Programs, *American Journal of Psychiatry,* **133**, 700–703.

Lowe, G. R. (1975) The Problem-Oriented System in a Multidisciplinary Psychiatric Milieu, *Canadian Psychiatric Association Journal,* **20**, 585–594.

Vickar, G. M. & Herjanic, M. (1976) The Use of Problem-Oriented Medical Records in Community Mental Health Centres, *American Journal of Psychiatry,* **133**, 340–341.

PATHOLOGY

Christie, R. W. (1973) The Problem-Oriented Autopsy Audit, *American Journal of Clinical Pathology,* **60**, 536–542.

Switz, D. M. (1976) The Problem-Oriented Medical Record: Evaluation and Management of Anaemia Before and During Use, *Archives of Internal Medicine,* **136**, 1119–1123.

Tasker, J. B. (1976) A Problem-Oriented Approach to Laboratory Diagnosis, *Veterinary Clinics of North America,* **6**, 515–522.

EDUCATION

Cross, H. D. (1970) Educational Needs as Determined by the Problem-Oriented Medical Record, *Journal of the Maine Medical Association,* **61**, 49–54.

Peck, R. L. (1972) Are Problem-Oriented Records the Key to House Staff Peer Review?, *Hospital Physician,* **8**, 46–48.

Margolis, C. Z., Sheehan, T. J. & Stickley, W. T. (1973) A Graded Problem-Oriented Record to Evaluate Clinical Performance, *Pediatrics,* **51**, 980–985.

Adamson, E. T. (1974) The Teaching and Use of the Problem-Oriented Medical Record in Medical Schools, *Journal of Medical Education,* **49**, 905–907.

Bashook, P. G., Sandlow, L. J. & Hammett, W. H. (1975) Education Plan Key to POMR Success, *Hospitals,* **49**, 54–58.

Bashook, P. G., Sandlow, L. J. & Hammett, W. H. (1975) Teaching Problem-Oriented Recording: A Systematic Approach, *Journal of Medical Education,* **50**, 959–964.

McIntyre, N. (1975) The Problem-Oriented Medical Record. Implications for Medical Education and Clinical Care, *Acta Clinica Belgica,* **30,** 343-348.

Thompson, S. P. (1975) Guidelines for Training Personnel in the Use of Problem Orientation, *League Exchange,* **103,** 9-14.

Wood, M. *et al,* (1975) A Systems Approach to Patient Care, Records, Curriculum, and Research in Family Practice, *Journal of Medical Education,* **50,** 1106-1112.

Barbaccia, J. C. (1976) Introducing Quality Assurance and Medical Audit into UCSF Medical Center Curriculum, *Journal of Medical Education,* **51,** 386-391.

Benbassat, J. & Schiffmann, A. (1976) An Approach to Teaching the Introduction to Clinical Medicine, *Annals of Internal Medicine,* **84,** 477-481.

Lloyd, G. J., Wyn Pugh, E. & McIntyre, N. (1976) The Problem-Orientated Medical Record and Its Educational Implications, *Medical Education,* **10,** 143-153.

Margolis, C. Z., Sheehan, T. J. & Meyers, A. (1976) Using a Workshop to Determine the Effectiveness of a Text on the Problem-Oriented Medical Record, *Journal of Medical Education,* **51,** 767-768.

Nelson, G. E., Graves, S. M., Holland, R. R., Nelson, J. M., Ratner, J. & Weed, L. L. (1976) A Performance-Based Method of Student Evaluation. *Medical Education,* **10,** 33-42.

Bouchard, R. E. & Tufo, H. M. (1977) A Dynamic Primary Care Curriculum Based on the Problem-Oriented System, *Journal of Medical Education,* **52,** 508-513.

NURSING

Field, F. W. (1971) Communication between Community Nurse and Physician: P.O.M.R. System Helps Clarity Patient Care Problems, *Nursing Outlook,* **19,** 722-725.

Bloom, J. T., Bressler, J., Kenney, M., Moldo, D. M. & Pardee, G. P. (1971) Problem-Orientated Charting, *American Journal of Nursing,* **71,** 2144-2148.

Schell, P. L. & Campbell, A. T. (1972) Problem-Oriented Medical Records: Not Just Another Way to Chart, *Nursing Outlook,* **20,** 510-514.

Thoma, D. & Pittman, K. (1972) Evaluation of Problems-Oriented Nursing Notes, *Journal of Nursing Administration,* **2,** 50-8.

Woody, M. & Mallison, M. (1973) The Problem-Oriented System for Patient Centred Care, *American Journal of Nursing,* **73,** 1168-1175.

Berni, R. (1975) Problem-Oriented Peer Review, *Nurse Practitioner,* **1,** 29-38.

McCloskey, J. C. (1975) The Problem-Oriented Record vs. the Nursing Care Plan: A Proposal, *Nursing Outlook,* **23,** 492-495.

VanMeter, M. J. & Scott, L. K. (1975) An Experience with Problem-Oriented Nursing Notes, *Journal of Neurosurgical Nursing,* **7,** 42-56.

Best, R., Bowen, G., Magill, K. & Morrell, C. (1976) POMR for Operating and Recovery Rooms, *Supervisory Nurse,* **7,** 18-22.

Kelly, M. E. & Roessler, L. M. (1976) Development of Interdisciplinary Problem-Oriented Recording in a Public Health Nursing Agency, *Journal of Nursing Administration,* **6,** 24-31.

Malloy, J. L. (1976) Taking Exception To Problem-Oriented Nursing Care, *American Journal of Nursing,* **76,** 582-583.

O'Connell, A. L. & Bates, B. (1976) The Case Method in Nurse Practitioner Education, *Nursing Outlook,* **24,** 243-246.

Woolley, F. R. & Kane, R. L. (1976) Telling It Like It Is Through Problem Orientation, *Nursing Care,* **9,** 25-27.

Wray, J. G. (1976) Problem-Oriented Recording in Community Nursing - A New Experience in Education, *International Journal of Nursing Studies,* **13,** 243-250.

Bacon, L. F. & Johnston, A. (1977) The Use of Problem-Oriented Record Prototypes, *Supervisory Nurse,* **8,** 30-31.

Hill, A. (1977) POR and Nursing Care Plans. Implementation of Nursing Process

O'Grady, T. P. (1977) Problem-Oriented Charting: The Educational and Implementation Challenge, *Supervisory Nurse*, **8**, 16–22.

MISCELLANEOUS

Dinsdale, S. M. & Mossman, P. L. (1970) Problem-Oriented Medical Record in Rehabilitation, *Archives of Physical Medicine and Rehabilitation*, **51**, 488–492.

Anderson, T. P. (1971) Problem-Orientation of Medical Records: Advantages in Long-Term Illness, *Postgraduate Medicine*, **50**, 274–277.

Milhous, R. L. (1972) Problem-Oriented Medical Record in Rehabilitation Management and Training, *Archives of Physical Medicine and Rehabilitation*, **53**, 182–185.

Potts, L. R. (1972) Problem-Oriented Record: Implications for Occupational Therapy, *American Journal of Occupational Therapy*, **26**, 288–291.

Crawford, G. B. (1973) The Problem-Oriented Medical Record in Long-Term Institutional Care, *Journal of the American Geriatrics Society*, **21**, 465–468.

Saitz, E. W. & Lewis, K. H. (1973) Use of the Problem-Oriented Medical Record by Junior Medical Staff in Paediatric Ambulatory Care, *Journal of Medical Education*, **48**, 453–455.

Voytovich, A. E. (1973) The Dietician/Nutritionist and the Problem-Oriented Medical Record i) The Physicians Viewpoint, *Journal of the American Dietetic Association*, **63**, 639–641.

Burger, C. S., Bjorn, J. C. & Cross, H. D. (1975) Problem-Oriented Pediatric Practice, *Current Problems in Paediatrics*, **5**, 29–44.

Dinsdale, S. M., Gent, M., Kline, G. & Milner, R. (1975) Problem-Oriented Medical Records: Their Impact on Staff Communication, Attitudes and Decision Making, *Archives of Physical Medicine and Rehabilitation*, **56**, 269–274.

Ingber, J. S. & Rose, L. F. (1975) The Problem-Oriented System. An Approach to Managing a Comprehensive Hospital Dental Service, *Dental Clinics of North America*, **19**, 703–715.

Ingber, J. S. & Rose, L. F. (1975) The Problem-Oriented Record: Clinical Application in a Teaching Hospital, *Journal of Dental Education*, **39**, 472–482.

Reinstein, L., Staas, W. E. Jr. & Marquette, C. H. (1975) A Rehabilitation Evaluation System which Complements the Problem-Oriented Medical Record, *Archives of Physical Medicine and Rehabilitation*, **56**, 396–399.

Worthley, L. I. (1975) A System-Structure Medical Record for Intensive Care Patient Documentation, *Critical Care Medicine*, **3**, 188–191.

Christie, R. W. (1976) Periodic Comprehensive Health Assessment and a Problem-Oriented Medical Record for Public School Students, *Journal of School Health*, **46**, 256–262.

Esterhay, R. J. Jr., Vogel, V. G., Fortner, C. L., Shapiro, H. M. & Wiernik, P. H. (1976) Cost Analysis of Leukemia Treatment: A Problem-Oriented Approach. *Cancer*, **37**, 646–652.

Tryon, A. F., Mann, W. V. & DeJong, N. (1976) Use of a Problem-Oriented Dental Record in Undergraduate Dental Education, *Journal of Dental Education*, **40**, 601–608.

Bouchard, M. M. & Shane, H. C. (1977) Use of the Problem-Oriented Medical Record in the Speech and Hearing Profession, *American Speech and Hearing Association*, **19**, 157–159.

Masters, L. E. (1977) Automated Medication List for Use with the Problem-Oriented Medical Record, *Journal of Family Practice*, **4**, 593–594.

Wingfield, W. E. & Stiff, M. (1977) Problem-Oriented Medical Records and the Cardiovascular System, *Veterinary Clinics of North America*, **7**, 227–239.

COMPUTERS

Schultz, J. R., Cantrill, S. V. & Morgan, K. G. (1971) An initial operational problem oriented medical record system – For storage, manipulation and retrieval of medical data, *AFIPS Conference Proceedings,* **38,** Montvale, N.J.: AFIPS Press.

Schultz, J. R. (1974) An Implementation Independent Description of a problem oriented medical information service: Philosophical principles and how they are used to define technological goals, *Digest of Papers, Micros and Minis Application and Design,* Compcon 74, September, Ninth Annual IEEE Computer Society International Conference.

Wanner, J. F. (1974) PROMIS, A Demanding Communications Problem, *NEREM 74 Record Part 1: Technical Papers.* IEEE, (66–69).

Brandejs, J. F., Kasowski, M. A. & Fortin, L. J. (1976) Information Systems. Part VII: Problem-Oriented Medical Records for Family Practice, *Canadian Medical Association Journal,* **114**(4), 371, 374, 384.

Oriented Medical Record at Karolinska Hospital – Format and Function, Users' Acceptance and Patient Attitude to Questionnaire, *Methods of Information in Medicine,* **15,** 11–20.

Meldman, M. J., Harris, D., Pellicore, R. J. & Johnson, E. L. (1977) A Computer-Assisted, Goal-Oriented Psychiatric Progress Note System, *American Journal Psychiatry,* **134**(1), 38–41.

Wakefield, J. S. & Yarnall, S. R. (1977) *Implementing the Problem-Oriented Medical Record.* Seattle: Medical Computer Services Association. (100 U-District Building, 1107 N.E. 45th Street, Seattle, Wash. 98105).

Index

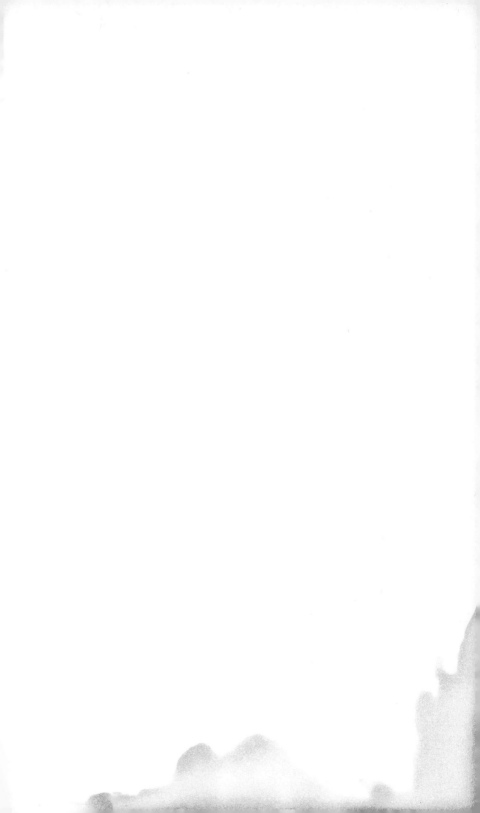